SEX

Also by Joe S. McIlhaney Jr., M.D.
1250 Health-Care Questions Women Ask

SEX

what you don't know can kill you

Joe S. McIlhaney Jr., M.D.
with Marion McIlhaney

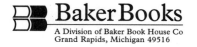

BakerBooks

A Division of Baker Book House Co
Grand Rapids, Michigan 49516

Some of the material in this book is based on Dr McIlhaney's previously published book, *Safe Sex* (1991).

Published by Baker Books
a division of Baker Book House Company
P.O. Box 6287, Grand Rapids, MI 49516-6287

Second printing, April 1997

Printed in the United States of America

Library of Congress Cataloging-in-Publication Data

McIlhaney, Joe S.
    Sex : what you don't know can kill you / Joe S. McIlhaney, with Marion McIlhaney.
      p. cm.
    ISBN 0-8010-5737-X
    1. Sexually transmitted diseases—Popular works. I. McIlhaney, Marion. II. Title.
    RC200.2.M35   1997
    616.95′1—dc20   ·   96-43362

The names of all the patients referred to in this book have been changed to protect their privacy.

To
Betty De Vries
for seeing value in my writings
for her gifts of confidence, counsel, and friendship

contents

Acknowledgments   9
Introduction   11
1. Sex—Powerful and Fragile   13

PART ONE   sexually transmitted diseases:
          symptoms and treatments

2. STDs—What Are They?   19
3. Chlamydia   23
4. Gonorrhea   30
5. Human Papillomavirus   34
6. Herpes   42
7. Syphilis   49
8. Hepatitis B   54
9. HIV/AIDS   57
10. Sexually Transmitted Vaginal Infections   65
11. Other Sexually Transmitted Diseases   70

PART TWO   sexual fulfillment:
          behaviors and risks

12. Mutual Masturbation, Outercourse, Dry Sex   79
13. Condoms   84
14. Mutual Monogamy: Cohabitation before Marriage   91
15. Uncommitted Sex and Emotional Health   94
16. Say No—Why and How   97
17. Secondary Virginity   104
18. 25, 35, 45—Still Single and Celibate?   108
19. Sexual Activity: Developing a Personal Code   114

acknowledgments

**tom smith, julie fontenot,
donna brinkley, rich tompkins,**
my co-workers
at the Medical Institute for Sexual Health
a team of competent and caring professionals
for their ideas, information, and encouragement

charlotte matthews
faithful friend, patient co-worker
the only person in the world
who can interpret my scribbles
and convert my notes into manuscript

lynne, anne, and caren
my daughters
joys of my life
for encouraging me to think through
and write about significant issues

marion
my wife
the love of my life
for reading and rereading
correcting, clarifying, and changing
improving the book

introduction

SEX–A WOW WORD, A STARTLING WORD! ALWAYS IT GRABS our attention. Images of sex are used by advertisers to sell everything from car parts to coffee. I'm not out to sell sex or use it to sell something else. My concern is to help you use this powerful force, to fit it into your overall sexuality as a man or woman, to have the greatest opportunity to achieve balance in your life now, and to enjoy freedom from regrets and life-threatening complications in the future.

Sex is perfectly good. As a matter of fact, it is great. Sex can bring enormous pleasure. Sex is physically and emotionally healthy if it is understood and used appropriately.

Unfortunately our society seems to be on a sexual binge. It has taken something wonderful and misused it, often with bitter, painful results. Individuals who exercise no control over their appetite for sex experience unfortunate consequences. We cannot indulge in sex binges without paying the price.

Those who thoughtlessly dive into sexual activity may find themselves swimming in a stew of sexually transmitted diseases, out-of-wedlock pregnancy, vaginal and penile discharge, abortions, medical procedures, medications, and on and on. Those who take the time to consider carefully their use of sex can almost be guaranteed freedom from all those problems.

That is what I want for you: life unencumbered by problems from the past, free of AIDS, free from regrets and flashbacks. I want you to be able to truly enjoy your life and your sexuality.

1

sex—powerful and fragile

DO YOU WANT TO HAVE A MAN LOVE YOU FOR EVERYTHING you are, not just for your body?

Do you want to eventually be married to a man who is tender toward you because he honestly cares about you?

Do you want to have children with him?

These are questions I have asked many of my younger patients. Every one of them, with shining eyes, answered these questions positively. Romance, joy, fun, and respectful treatment by a man are legitimate ideals that inspire women. These same notions also draw men to relationships.

Men do not relish relationships with one woman after another, like a bee going from flower to flower. That is a myth. The truth is that, in general, men are sifting through their women friends, looking for that one special person with whom to settle down.

If this is true, why are so many of my young patients having sexual intercourse? Why do these same girls say that *all* their high school friends or *all* their college friends are having sex? A new patient, a twenty-one-year-old, certainly thought that. She started having sex when she was fourteen. By the time I saw her, she had had eight or ten partners. Changing partners, to her, was no big deal.

Maybe the conventional wisdom is wrong. Maybe people are different now that we are about to close the twentieth century. Maybe women don't care whether sex is packaged with

13

love. Maybe having sexual intercourse with one man this year and another man next year is really satisfying. Maybe men are really just animals–like an unneutered male dog that takes off after a female the second he gets a whiff that she is in heat.

Maybe, but I doubt it.

Men and women of all ages are more than animals driven purely by instinct. They have an inborn desire for something more than purely animalistic acts. Their yearnings for joy, romance, dignity, and the ability to protect themselves from peril now so that they can have a better future are there–although they may be deeply buried.

> If we focus only on the sex act and ignore the relationship between two people that makes sex human, we destroy the fragile side of sex.

If you doubt that, take a good look at yourself. Deep down in your inner being you want to be treated with love and respect. You enjoy that. And you enjoy the thought of treating another person the same way. If you take time to think about it, the honest truth is that eventually you probably do want to have a wife or husband and your own family.

Why all this confusion about sex, relationships between men and women, love, and romance? Could it be that while we realize how special to our humanity sex is, we allow the powerful, more animalistic drive to have sexual intercourse to eclipse the fragile and human part of sex?

Sexual intercourse is both powerful and delicate at the same time–an amazing fact! Because sex is such a powerful drive, we may think bad things cannot happen to it or come from it. Nothing could be further from the truth. If we focus only on the sex act and ignore the relationship between two people that makes sex human, we destroy the fragile side of sex. When we destroy that relational, fragile side of sex, we take the risk of destroying what sex should be to a human being–the deepest form of communication between two people who love each other. All that is left is a brutish act that soon grows wearisome.

It is futile to seek to rekindle the fire of sexual excitement by finding a new partner. The cycle of disappointment is repeated and the result is more disillusionment and emotional burden and baggage.

A good illustration compares sex to fire. Fire is both good and bad. Fire is certainly good when it is used to cook food or to keep ourselves warm. But fire can burn, scar, and kill when it gets out of control. One of my patients was with her husband in a sailboat when the cook top exploded, throwing fuel all over them and setting them on fire. If they had not leaped into the water, they would have been killed. They will carry the scars on their bodies for the rest of their lives. Is fire good or bad? We all know that depends on how it is used.

Sex is the same: both good and bad, depending on how we use it. Most things in life are like this. Chocolate is fine, unless we eat too much of it. Then chocolate can make us very sick.

Driving a car is a good thing. Most people do it. It brings pleasure and gives us a lot of mobility. If driving is so good, why did it turn out so bad for a couple of young boys—not old enough to drive—who stole a car and were killed in a crash? Our local paper reported that these boys tried to drive without following the guidelines that make driving a good and healthy activity. Almost daily newspapers report deaths of those who drive inappropriately.

When sex is misused, it causes people to grow emotionally hardened as they flit from one sex partner to another sex partner. The path they are following is most likely strewn with potential damage to their bodies. Damage could include infertility, viral infections that can cause cancer, and even HIV infection.

All human activity must follow the rules. The young men who drove the car would have had much less risk of calamity if they had waited until they had taken driver's training, obtained their licenses, and driven by the rules.

Driving is a simple activity when compared to sexual activity, but it does have some appropriate parallels. There are great dangers when one begins sexual activity at too young an age. There are "rules" that can help to avoid the risks of sexually transmitted diseases and out-of-wedlock pregnancies. These rules will be discussed in later chapters.

Sexuality is an integral part of one's humanity—and that involves more than sexual intercourse—it includes "womanness" or "man-ness." Sexual intercourse is just one part of sexuality. And sexuality is only one part of one's humanity. It is not necessary to have sexual intercourse to experience one's full sexuality or humanity as either a man or as a woman. To help bring a balanced understanding of what it means to be a man or woman in the fullest sense, many of the complicated aspects surrounding the subject of sexual intercourse will be faced head-on in later chapters.

PART ONE

sexually transmitted diseases

symptoms and treatments

2

STDs—what are they?

WHAT IS A SEXUALLY TRANSMITTED DISEASE OR AN STD? SIMply stated, it is an infection that is passed from one person to another during sexual activity. Some years ago a common term for sexually transmitted diseases was VD or venereal disease.

Body fluids and secretions are exchanged between partners during intimate sexual contact. The exchange occurs not only during vaginal intercourse but also during other activity, such as oral sex and "outercourse."

If an individual has a sexually transmitted disease, some of the germs are in that person's body fluids. Most STD germs are very fragile. They require warmth and moisture and are susceptible to temperature change, sunlight, and other conditions that exist outside the body. Inside the warm, moist body, however, STD germs are extremely potent and can cause permanent damage. In the case of AIDS, the germs become a monster that kills.

Thankfully, most STD germs cannot live long outside the human body and are not normally exchanged when people hug or shake hands. Neither are STDs transmitted by using the same computer, telephone, toilet seat, or tools that an infected person uses.

STDs in women

Vaginal intercourse is the most common way for a woman to become infected with an STD. If a woman is infected with an STD vaginally, her vaginal secretions and often vulvar and vaginal tissues will contain these germs. If a man is infected, usually his semen and often the skin of his penis and scrotum will contain the disease-causing organisms.

During vaginal intercourse a woman's vagina is a receptacle for the teaspoon of semen a man normally ejaculates. If the man has an STD, his ejaculate can infect the vagina and from there the germs can be passed into a woman's bloodstream, as occurs with HIV. Studies indicate that material deposited in the vagina shows up twenty minutes later in the uterus and fallopian tubes.

STDs in men

Even though a man is not a receptacle for fluid in the sense that a woman is, he can contract an STD through vaginal intercourse because his penis acts like a miniature vacuum cleaner. It will suction minute amounts of secretions from the woman's vagina into his urethra (the tube in the penis through which urine and semen flow). If the woman has a vaginal STD, during intercourse the germs can be drawn up into a man's reproductive organs where they can cause infection.

Vaginal intercourse is not the only way to transmit STDs; any intimate sexual contact can transmit infections. Disease agents from a partner's genital area may be transmitted to the mouth of a sex partner during oral sex. Anal sex can result in an STD of the rectum.

Some STD organisms, such as herpes and HPV, can infect moist genital skin if the infected skin of one person touches the uninfected skin of a sex partner, even though they do not have penetrative sex.

permanent effects of STDs

Sex is good. But when sex is used inappropriately in a way that produces hurt, it can totally change the future course of one's life. Do not plan on a second chance to undo the hurt. There may not be a second chance.

> STD germs are extremely potent and can cause permanent damage. Even one unwise sexual encounter can change your life forever.

If a woman gets a pelvic infection, that infection may leave scars that can make her infertile. Nothing can be done to make those infection sites normal again. If a woman becomes infected with HIV, she can never become uninfected, and will probably die from that infection.

We often assume that if we make a mistake it can always be corrected and life will become normal again. That may be a wrong assumption in the area of sexuality and sexually transmitted diseases. True, to become pregnant a woman may be able to have an in vitro fertilization procedure done if she is badly scarred from a pelvic infection. But she does not have a guarantee that it will be successful and there are costly medical bills to pay for even an unsuccessful procedure.

Consider a young patient of mine who had intercourse when she was eighteen and as a result developed pelvic inflammatory disease (PID), caused by a chlamydia infection. All of her pelvic organs were scarred, as though glue had been poured on the fallopian tubes, ovaries, and intestines. The result was pain: pain with bowel movements, pain with working out, and pain with intercourse. She had pain year after year. Finally at age twenty-four, the pain was so severe that she had to have her uterus, tubes, and ovaries removed. The woman had never been married and never had a baby. Now she never will. An extreme case? About 75 percent of women who have PID will eventually need some type of medical treatment. Often these women have surgery to help them become fertile enough to have a baby. Only 30 percent of these surgical procedures are successful enough to enable a woman to become pregnant.

Another patient of mine, a forty-five-year-old woman, had been married but divorced. She allowed a man she had known for fifteen years to have intercourse with her. She came to my office in tears because she had a herpes infection. Now she feels contaminated and sexually unattractive as month after month she continues to experience the herpes outbreaks.

A nineteen-year-old had a very small venereal wart at the opening of her vagina. She was devastated and could not believe that she had become infected with an STD by her friend who never mentioned that he had warts on his penis.

These people will probably be affected by these diseases for years, perhaps for a lifetime. So may you, if you become infected. Even one unwise sexual encounter can change your life forever. I have seen firsthand the damaged and destroyed lives STDs have caused. Most of the time there is no second chance. The epidemic is dangerous and deadly. It has permeated our culture.

Sexually transmitted diseases are transmitted by having sex with an infected partner. If you are saving sex for that long-term protected relationship with a mate who is not infected—marriage—relax and do not worry about STDs. Enjoy the freedom and safety that is yours.

3

chlamydia

ABOUT 4 MILLION PEOPLE IN THE U.S. DEVELOP A NEW
CHLAMYDIA INFECTION EACH YEAR.

BETWEEN 8 AND 25% OF SEXUALLY ACTIVE COLLEGE STU-
DENTS HAVE CHLAMYDIA.

APPROXIMATELY 31% OF PATIENTS EXAMINED IN SEXUALLY
TRANSMITTED DISEASE CENTERS HAVE CHLAMYDIA.

CHLAMYDIA IS THE MOST COMMON BACTERIAL STD IN THE UNITED
States, and teenagers have the highest chlamydia infection
rate of any group. A woman usually receives the bacteria
from a man during intercourse. She can carry it in her cervix,
uterus, tubes, and ovaries for months or years and not know
it. When it does flare up, it causes pain: pelvic pain, painful
intercourse, and painful bowel movements. Often a woman
will also have a fever and urethral discharge. One of the usually unavoidable, serious results is infertility.

A dangerous feature of chlamydia is that a person can be
infected for days or years and not be aware of it. Most studies say that 70 percent of the people who carry chlamydia
have no symptoms. The disease can be transmitted during
intercourse without either partner knowing it. Frequent
changing of sex partners results in a rampaging, silent cycle
of infection.

A new patient of mine was married for a year when she
came in for a check-up. She had been a virgin when she mar-

ried but her husband had had many sex partners before they met. The couple made a decision not to have intercourse until they were married. Her husband had been tested for sexually transmitted diseases before they were married and the test results showed no infections.

In spite of these precautions, I encouraged my patient to be tested for chlamydia and gonorrhea because test results from men can be unreliable. Her test results were positive. She had been infected with these germs for the entire year of her marriage without any symptoms. What worried both of us is the possibility that some of the germs may have damaged her fallopian tubes. We won't know for certain until they stop using contraception.

Why didn't the husband's premarital test for STDs reveal the presence of the germs? Often STD tests on males are inaccurate because the urethra is dry and it is uncomfortable to have a swab put into the end of the penis. I recommend that a male who has had sexual intercourse in the past have two tests done for both chlamydia and gonorrhea before he has intercourse with a new female partner. That is the only way he can be sure he is not going to pass germs to her. A few weeks after the couple begins to have intercourse, I recommend that she also be tested for chlamydia and gonorrhea, just to be completely sure she is free of infection.

chlamydia in women

infertility

A patient came to me for an in vitro fertilization procedure. She had been married for three years and was unable to become pregnant. Her doctor found that her tubes were completely blocked. She had had multiple sex partners in the past but had never had pelvic pain or discomfort. She did not know that her tubes had become infected, probably by chlamydia, and that she had become sterile.

Infertility, the inability to become pregnant, is a terrible burden for a couple. In the United States today the most rapidly increasing cause of female infertility is chlamydia infection of reproductive organs. Chlamydia infections cause pus, and when this infection develops in a woman's tubes and ovaries, it is as though glue has been poured over these delicate tissues. The tissues stick together and form scar. The scar tissue damages the sensitive organs. They will never again be normal. For example, the tiny hairlike projections (cilia) in the inner part of the fallopian tubes normally sweep an egg from the ovaries down the tube. When the cilia are destroyed or damaged by scarring, it is impossible for the egg to be swept from the ovary into the uterus, where a new life can begin.

Chlamydia lives inside cells and is half bacteria and half virus. About 70 percent of the people who carry chlamydia have no symptoms.

Usually the infection, pain, and scarring, called pelvic inflammatory disease (PID), is caused by chlamydia. Occasionally it may be the result of gonorrhea. A PID infection is one of the worst threats to a woman's fertility. One episode of chlamydia PID can result in a 25 percent chance of infertility. Since there is no immunity from chlamydia, a second infection could result in as high as a 50 percent chance of infertility. Surgery or in vitro fetilization may be done, but even these procedures cannot guarantee a pregnancy and they are very expensive, often uncomfortable, and extremely stressful.

A few years ago, a high school student was referred to me by her family doctor. She had been sexually active with a "big man on campus" who had infected her with both chlamydia and human papillomavirus (HPV). The doctor had treated her for venereal warts and for a year tried to eliminate her abdominal pain that he had diagnosed as being caused by gonorrhea. When I saw her I found that chlamydia was the cause of her pain and after appropriate antibiotic treatment, the pain finally left. The saddest part of this case history is that the young woman probably has serious scarring of her fallopian tubes and ovaries because the PID infection had been present so long. For more than a year pus was poured over her sensitive internal tissues. She will probably be infertile. Of course, by the time I saw the patient, her boyfriend had moved on to other girls and no doubt passed the infections on to them.

tubal pregnancy

Infertility, unfortunately, is not the only result of PID. If a woman's tube is only partially scarred, she may conceive but have a tubal (ectopic) pregnancy. The egg may be blocked from reaching the uterus, but sperm, which are smaller and can move on their own, may reach the egg that is trapped in the fallopian tube and fertilize it. A fallopian tube is too small to hold a pregnancy and after three or four weeks it may rupture. The resulting hemorrhage can be dangerous—in fact, tubal pregnancies are the leading cause of death among pregnant teenagers. If a woman's first pregnancy is an ectopic pregnancy, she has a 75 percent chance of being sterile. An ectopic pregnancy is evidence that a woman's fallopian tubes may be abnormal because of either PID or some other problem.

A young, unmarried, sexually active patient of mine went to college in another city. She called one day to say that she was pregnant and having abdominal pain, and her doctors thought she needed surgery for a probable tubal pregnancy. I told her she needed the surgery. I did not have the heart to tell her that since this was her first pregnancy and it was ectopic, there was a good chance she might be sterile. That was several years ago. She eventually did marry. She and her husband have been trying for two years now to become pregnant. Unfortunately she is probably sterile. All this heartache because she thought it was okay to have sex with a couple of guys while she was in college.

chlamydia in men

As many as 70 percent of infected men have no symptoms of a chlamydia infection and they can unknowingly infect their sex partners. Symptoms might include a discharge of pus from the penis and burning sensations with urination. Chlamydia infects the internal genital organs: the urethra, the prostate, and the seminal vesicles. Epididymitis can develop, which, if not properly treated, can result in infertility. Even though this infertility can usually be reversed with antibiotics, it is not pleasant for a man to be infected. Fear, guilt of possibly infecting others, a regime of tests, and medications, are part of the experience of a male being treated for chlamydia.

A more unusual complication in males is Reiter's syndrome, a painful systemic illness. There is a 50 percent chance of a patient with Reiter's syndrome being a urethral carrier of chlamydia.

Male homosexuals can develop rectal chlamydia infections. Having oral sex with an infected person can result in a throat infection from chlamydia being passed on to future sex partners through oral sex.

diagnosing chlamydia

To test a woman for chlamydia, the doctor would need to do a pelvic examination and test secretions from the cervix. To test a man for chlamydia, the doctor would put a swab into the end of the penis (the urethra) for a short distance and test the secretions for chlamydia and gonorrhea. Studies suggest that men may carry chlamydia deep in their internal genital organs without testing positive for it, and yet be able to pass it on to someone else.

It is possible for a woman to have chlamydia in her fallopian tubes and yet have a negative test from her cervical secretions. The only way a woman with this situation would know she was carrying chlamydia would be for her to have a laparoscopy for direct testing of her fallopian tubes. Under general anesthesia an optical telescope (laparoscope) is put through a small incision in the edge of the umbilicus to view the fallopian tubes. The surgeon can then swab the fallopian tubes or take a small pinch from the tip of the tube to test for chlamydia.

treating chlamydia

Chlamydia is a weird germ. It is half bacteria and half virus. It lives inside cells. It is often accompanied by gonorrhea and many doctors will treat a patient for both germs if she has PID. If a man or woman tests positive for chlamydia but has no pain or symptoms, a physician may treat that patient with either tetracycline or a new drug, azithromycin (Zithromax). This usually clears up such a simple infection. The problem with treating chlamydia this way is that although the drug may eliminate the infection in a woman's cervical area, she may still have the infection in her fallopian tubes. An estimated 20 percent of women who have had the tetracycline treatment are left with the infection in their fallopian tubes. If a woman has no symptoms, pain, or pelvic discomfort after treatment, it is unlikely that she and her doctor will pursue the more aggressive laparoscopic testing of the fallopian tubes. All the while, though undetected, a low-grade smoldering infection may still be present. This is a frustrating problem that seems to have no full solution.

It is extremely important to treat the woman's sex partner for chlamydia while she is undergoing treatment, even if he has no symptoms. If he is not treated, he can reinfect her as soon as she stops taking antibiotics.

The woman who has actually developed PID as a result of chlamydia or gonorrhea must have much more intensive treatment, which may include hospitalization and intravenous antibiotics.

long-term effects of chlamydia

Chlamydia infections can be devastating for a woman. Scarring of fallopian tubes is the culprit in many cases of infertility. Chlamydia is also often the culprit in an ectopic or tubal pregnancy. Untreated chlamydia is often the cause of uterine infection during the first few days after delivery. A baby has about a 66 percent chance of becoming infected during the birth process if the mother has chlamydia. Babies can develop eye infections, pneumonia, or inner ear infections. These chronic ear infections can prevent a baby from developing good language skills and listening abilities, which could cause later learning problems.

4

gonorrhea

ABOUT 80% OF MEN AND WOMEN INFECTED WITH GON-
ORRHEA ARE UNAWARE OF ITS PRESENCE FOR VARYING
LENGTHS OF TIME.

BETWEEN 20 AND 40% OF PEOPLE WHO HAVE GONORRHEA
ALSO HAVE CHLAMYDIA.

ONE BOUT OF GONORRHEA PID INFECTION IN A WOMAN RE-
SULTS IN A 12% POSSIBILITY OF INFERTILITY; A SECOND
BOUT OF SUCH INFECTION RESULTS IN A 25% POSSIBILITY
OF INFERTILITY.

GONORRHEA INFECTIONS HAVE PLAGUED HUMANS FOR THOU-
sands of years. Since the days of Aristotle, gonorrhea has
plagued rich and poor, peasants and kings. Just because it
has been around for so long does not mean that it is a trivial
problem. It is a terrible affliction for those who become infected with it. Although it is quite similar to the chlamydia
germ, gonorrhea has some insidious differences.

Almost never transmitted by any way other than intercourse, gonorrhea is caused by pus-producing bacteria. Like
chlamydia, it may infect a person for days or months without any symptoms. It is highly communicable. There is a 40
percent chance of contracting gonorrhea from just one sex
act with an infected individual. Teens are especially susceptible to the disease and the number of teens infected with it
is rising alarmingly.

In addition to initially being a no-symptom disease, gonorrhea can be an extremely dangerous disease. Occasionally

men and women can pass gonorrhea into the bloodstream and then into a joint. This results in septic arthritis, an infection that requires intensive antibiotic therapy. It can leave a permanent scar in a joint.

A colleague of mine, an orthopedist, saw a fifteen-year-old girl who had a severely infected knee joint. He inserted a needle in the joint to remove the pus. Tests revealed that the infection was caused by gonorrhea. Although the girl was still a virgin, she had had "dry sex" (genital contact without penetration). Evidently germs in her partner's secretions spilled on her external genital organs and then made their way up her vaginal canal into her body. The gonorrhea germ had gone into her bloodstream to the knee joint. She thought her limited sexual behavior eliminated the risk of infection. She was wrong.

gonorrhea in women

Often one of the first indications that a woman has an infection caused by gonorrhea is a burning sensation with urination and a puslike discharge from the urethra. Although the infection may cause the need to urinate frequently, it may also make urination painful or impossible. Then catherization is necessary.

If the Bartholin's glands, which provide secretions and moisture for a woman's vulva, become infected, the glands can swell, become abscessed, or develop cysts which show up as a painful swelling near the lower opening of the vagina. This is an extremely uncomfortable problem and brings many patients to doctors' offices. The abscesses can be opened under local anesthetic, usually bringing temporary relief. The problem is that if the opening closes down (and this happens often), another abscess or cyst can develop in the same location. This can recur for months or years.

Gonorrhea can also infect the uterus, fallopian tubes, and ovaries. If this occurs, it is called pelvic inflammatory disease (PID). Pus produced by this infection can cause tubes, ovaries, and intestines to stick together, just as happens with chlamydia. The infection can also create pockets of pus (abscesses) in the pelvis. Fallopian tubes are often scarred shut, causing infertility. Although PID is more often caused by chlamydia, gonorrhea is still a common cause.

gonorrhea in men

Although men infected with gonorrhea may not notice any problems for some time, the first symptoms are often burning sensations during urination and the need to urinate frequently. Another symptom can be a fairly heavy, puslike discharge from the penis.

Men can develop scarring of the urethra (the tube in the penis through which urine and semen pass). If the tube becomes blocked by scars, urination becomes impossible and painful dilatations must be done. If the scarring is severe, plastic surgery may be needed to rebuild a urethra to allow urination and ejaculation.

general symptoms of gonorrhea

Both men and women can develop rectal infections from gonorrhea if they have anal intercourse. Symptoms include diarrhea, pus in the stool, painful bowel movements, and irritation of the anus.

Gonorrhea-infected people who engage in oral sex may spread the infection to the mouth and throat of their partner.

Other symptoms of gonorrhea infection include high fever, skin rashes, and even arthritis. Hospitalization may be required to treat stubborn infections.

diagnosing gonorrhea

If gonorrhea is suspected, the secretions from a man's penis or from a woman's cervix or vagina are gathered and cultured. If the gonococci bacteria grow, the diagnosis is made. Most doctors culture patients for chlamydia and gonorrhea at the same time because from 20 to 40 percent of patients having one disease also have both infections.

treating gonorrhea

A major concern is that strains of gonorrhea resistant to penicillin have been found in all fifty states. Therefore a drug called ceftriaxone (Rocephin) or one of the newer cephalo-sporin antibiotics is usually prescribed. These antibiotics cost about ten times as much as penicillin. Some gonorrhea strains have even become resistant to the newer antibiotics. A person could be treated with an antibiotic that is not effective against a specific strain of gonorrhea and the infection would not be controlled. Infection would then continue, allowing further damage to occur until the antibiotic is changed. A woman's tubes might be irreversibly damaged by the time an effective antibiotic is found.

> Strains of gonorrhea resistant to penicillin have been found in all fifty states.

If a woman develops pelvic inflammatory disease, she may need to be hospitalized for intensive antibiotic therapy.

Newborns can pick up the gonorrhea organism in the birth canal if their mothers have the infection. All newborns in the United States now routinely have their eyes washed with a 2 percent silver nitrate solution. The solution kills any gonococci present. When this is not done, blindness often occurs.

Gonorrhea is a sexually transmitted disease, spread by having intercourse with an infected person. If you are saving sex for marriage, relax and do not worry about gonorrhea. Enjoy the freedom and safety that is yours in not being exposed to this terrible infection.

5

human papillomavirus

HPV IS THE MOST COMMON SEXUALLY TRANSMITTED DISEASE.

APPROXIMATELY 33 TO 45% OF SEXUALLY ACTIVE SINGLE PEOPLE ARE INFECTED WITH HPV, OFTEN WITHOUT SYMPTOMS FOR MANY MONTHS.

UP TO 70% OF FEMALE HPV VICTIMS WILL LATER DEVELOP PRECANCEROUS CHANGES OF THE CERVIX (SOME WILL EVEN DEVELOP CERVICAL CANCER).

A 40% INCREASE IN VULVAR CANCER (USUALLY CAUSED BY HPV) IN CONNECTICUT HAS OCCURRED IN THE LAST 30 YEARS, ACCORDING TO A RECENT STUDY.

HUMAN PAPILLOMAVIRUS (HPV) IS EXTREMELY COMMON, dangerous, and aggravating. You may be familiar with the pesky venereal warts (condyloma) it causes. HPV infections are the most common medical reason American women in the reproductive age of life see their gynecologists.

Human papillomavirus grows best in moist areas of the body. It is commonly a genital growth that grows better in women than in men, often growing in the vagina or on the cervix of women. The virus is mixed in with the sexual secretions of men and women and can grow on moist skin. That is why it is so easily spread even by genital contact that does not include penetrative sex. That is also why it is not usually contained by condoms. Most experts agree that condoms do little to protect against this, the most common STD.

There are over seventy different strains. Human papillomavirus types 6, 11, 16, 18, 31, 33, and 35 are the culprits that usually cause venereal warts and cancerous and precancerous changes of the genitals of both men and women.

Either you or your partner can have HPV without being aware of it. Studies indicate that the communicable period for symptomless HPV may last for many months. Even though you or your partner have no symptoms of HPV, the virus is easily transmitted by sexual activity, with or without penetration.

HPV in women

A couple of years ago I treated a patient with a small dime-size area of warts. I treated her with the usual podophyllin, but after several treatments she still had the warts. Several times I used an acid application (TCA). Still no success. So I surgically removed them. They grew back. Her sex partner saw his doctor two or three times but he didn't have warts. They stopped having sex for several months. The warts persisted. Finally, I used the laser not only to burn away the warts, but also to lightly burn her entire vulvar area. This finally stopped her wart problem. Emotional turmoil, expensive medical care, and interruption of a relationship were part of the price demanded of her to get rid of her warts. These were small warts, but they were not a small problem. Not for her.

> Genital HPV has a particular affinity for young women. Condoms do little to protect against this common STD.

During pregnancy venereal warts tend to proliferate quite rapidly and become quite large. A pregnant teenager was referred to me because of huge venereal warts, bigger than my two fists. The surgical procedure to remove the warts took over two hours. Unfortunately, the warts grew back and became so large that they obstructed her vagina and made a cesarean section necessary.

Human papillomavirus can cause far worse trouble than warts. Only in the past few years have medical experts realized another fact about HPV infection. Almost all abnormal Pap smears indicating precancerous or cancerous cells are a result of infection from HPV. This is the primary reason doctors advise every woman to have a Pap smear every year. Studies on women with premalignant or malignant Pap smear results indicate that between 63 and 80 percent of their current male partners had venereal warts on their penis.

An abnormal Pap smear usually means more tests, all of which are explained in the section on treating human papillomavirus. Unfortunately, the necessary tests may weaken the cervix, which may contribute to a premature baby if a woman later becomes pregnant. This means that if she becomes infected with HPV, she can develop a precancer. The precancerous condition can usually be treated and cleared but that might leave her with a weakened cervix. A weakened cervix can cause her to have a premature baby with resulting problems—a string of events never anticipated when this person decided to have sex years ago.

But that is not all an HPV infection can do. It can cause precancerous changes in skin cells of the penis, the vagina, and the vulva. If such cells are not treated, they can eventually change into invasive cancer.

Although cervical cancer is the primary danger from HPV, about 10 percent of women with cervical cancer will eventually develop cancer of the vulva. If vulvar cancer is extensive, the entire vulvar area must usually be removed.

Vestibulitis is another problem that may be associated with HPV. Most specialists believe HPV causes some cases of vestibulitis (irritation of the tissues at the entrance to the vagina), even though recent evidence indicates that it may not be the primary culprit. Vestibulitis is a terrible problem for a woman. It can ruin her sex life for years.

This happened to a twenty-four-year-old patient of mine. She was a virgin who let an older, very sexually experienced man have intercourse with her. Within weeks she developed such severe vulvar burning that she could no longer tolerate intercourse. Even though she stopped having intercourse, she continued to have intermittent severe burning of the vulva. After a few months the man left her because of her inability to have intercourse.

Babies born to women who have HPV in their genital tracts may later develop warts of the larynx. Often multiple surgical procedures are necessary to remove these recurring warts. The procedures can cause permanent scarring of the baby's vocal cords. Although this problem is uncommon, it does occur.

Genital HPV has a particular affinity for young women. During the teenage years bodies seem to be more susceptible to this disease than during adulthood. For example, in one study, an evaluation of nearly 800,000 Pap smears of women of all ages revealed that nearly one-fourth of the abnormal smears were from women between the ages of fifteen and nineteen. Most of these teenagers had sexual intercourse before the age of fifteen. More than half had more than one partner. Susceptibility of teenage bodies to this infection coupled with sex at a young age with multiple partners seems to lead directly to a high rate of infection.

A seventeen-year-old girl came to my office because an exam at a Planned Parenthood Clinic revealed either a lump or a wart on her cervix. It was indeed a wart. She told me she had had intercourse with three people. However, during the previous year, she had intercourse with only one man. She remembered that a previous boyfriend had noticed some lumps on his penis but had dismissed them as being unimportant.

HPV in men

The primary risk for men who have HPV is the danger of cancer of the penis, although this is not a common occurrence.

Almost all penile cancer is the result of HPV. If a man de-velops a wartlike growth on his penis or scrotum, he needs to get a diagnosis and treatment soon.

diagnosing human papillomavirus infection

One of the biggest problems with diagnosing a genital HPV infection is that it can be undetected for a long time. The virus may be in a woman's vagina without developing into a wart or producing an abnormal Pap smear. Recent tests indicate that from 10 to 46 percent of otherwise healthy women may have dormant HPV.

In men the presence of HPV may be undetected because men's external genitalia are dry and if there are any warts, they may be small and almost undetectable.

In men, warts caused by HPV usually develop on the penis, scrotum, or sometimes in or around the anus. The warts are very contagious. About 85 percent of women whose regular sex partners have these warts will develop similar growths within eight months.

In women, warts caused by HPV usually appear in the groin, on the vulva, in the vagina, on the cervix, or in and around the anus.

Even if a person does not have warts or precancer or can-cer, doctors can detect the presence of HPV by doing a DNA test. The most common test kit is Virapap HPV DNA De-tection Kit. A swab of the woman's vagina or of a man's pe-nile or scrotal areas is taken. If there are no warts present and no precancer developing, there is no treatment for the pres-ence of HPV. Therefore there seems to be no reason to have an HPV DNA test just because one has had sexual activity with a partner who might have HPV.

Human papillomavirus infection causes warts in other parts of the human body. Although the strains of HPV that cause warts on hands and feet do not normally infect the genital area, recent evidence suggests that parents or adult healthcare workers can pass HPV from warts on their fingers and hands to the genital organs of babies or children while taking care of them. The frequency with which this actually occurs is still not known.

treating human papillomavirus

When a patient goes to a doctor because he or she has small wartlike genital growths, the doctor may perhaps use a magnifying instrument called a colposcope to examine them. The suspicious area may be stained with dilute acetic acid, a vinegar-type acid that makes the warts more visible. For women the areas involved will probably be the vulva, vagina, and/or cervix. For men the involved areas are usually the groin, penis, and/or scrotum.

A small portion of the growth may be removed for laboratory testing (biopsy) if there is any question about its identity. No doctor would want to treat a growth as a mere wart when it might already be a cancer.

If a woman's Pap smear indicates precancerous or cancerous changes, a colposcopy of the cervix will usually be done. This involves staining the cervix with dilute acetic acid for a few minutes and then magnifying the area with the colposcope. Small biopsies would be taken to make certain that the HPV had not already caused cancer.

If invasive cancer is not present, a conization procedure (removal of a small cone-shaped wedge of tissue) is done. This procedure is most often done under local anesthetic but a patient may elect to have a general anesthetic. An alternate treatment (LEEP procedure) is to pass a small, hot wire through the cervix to cut the area containing the abnormal cells. This is usually performed under local anesthetic. A pathologist checks to see if all abnormal cells have been removed and if any cancer is present. If the growth is cancer, it must usually be treated aggressively with radical surgery or radiation therapy.

If the Pap smear continues to be abnormal, all the procedures need to be repeated periodically until the Pap smear stays normal.

If venereal warts are present, podophyllin or trichloracetic acid are used to treat them. Multiple treatments are often necessary. If the acid treatments are not successful, freezing the warts, using the laser, or cutting away the warts can be tried. If the warts persist, multiple injections of interferon may be tried. This is very expensive but can sometimes eliminate resistant warts.

Venereal warts may disappear after the simplest treatment, but for some men and women the aggravation can require many years of treatment and thousands of dollars in medical fees.

A man contacted me by phone recently and vented his frustration about penile warts he had had for years. They had persisted in spite of all the treatments listed above: laser, acid, surgery, cryosurgery. Discouraged, depressed, and angry, he was beginning to feel that he should never be married because he dreaded passing HPV to his wife.

All this aggravation could have been prevented . . . if only!

The answer to avoiding HPV is not condoms. Condoms give almost no protection against HPV. It is a skin-to-skin disease that has no reliable prevention—except one: abstinence until marriage.

Today some specialists say that once a person has HPV, he or she will always carry the virus. No one knows for sure, but that uncertainty is not important. If you have warts, you need treatment until they disappear. If you have an abnormal Pap smear, you need treatment until the Pap smear stays normal. If you have no more warts and your Pap smear stays normal, your future husband will almost certainly not contract an HPV infection from you. So what difference does it make if you carry the virus the rest of your life provided it does not ever cause you or your partner any difficulty?

A woman sent me a letter after reading one of my books. This is the gist of what she said.

> I was promiscuous for sixteen years. I entered into many sexual relationships, and, as a result, I acquired human papillomavirus. I was diagnosed with it in 1987 and had treatment for it. My problem is that now I've met a man in my church and we have been dating. I think he is the one I would like to marry. But, remembering my HPV situation, I am mortified about it. There is no way to get around the embarrassment of telling him about it eventually, but it is not something I look forward to. I am thinking that I would just rather forget the thought of marrying and resolve to live a celibate life rather than live with the guilt and shame of possibly infecting my husband.

I tried to reassure her that since she has had no warts for several years, she is unlikely to pass the virus to her husband. But even if he does get warts, he could have them treated and probably be okay. She can probably live a normal life without medical problems from HPV. No guarantees, though.

Choose not to have intercourse with anyone except the one person you select to live with for the rest of your life. Even if that person has previously contracted HPV, the two of you are safer if you stay together and don't have sex with anyone else the rest of your lives. There are more than seventy different strains of HPV and recent evidence shows that the fewer number of strains of this virus you are exposed to, the safer you are.

6

herpes

It is possible to contract herpes from an infected person even when no sore is present.

People who develop herpes in the genital area often continue to have outbreaks for the rest of their lives.

There is no medical cure for the herpes virus.

When I first began my medical practice, I worked at the University of Texas Student Health Center for a while to help augment my income. As a specialist, I would see the patients with more severe gynecologic problems.

A coed came in one day. She could hardly walk, had a fever and chills, ached all over, and had such terrible sores on her vulvar area that she would not allow herself to urinate because it burned so badly. A few days before her symptoms began, she had intercourse with a rock star who played on campus. I put her in the hospital, put a catheter into her bladder, and started her on medication for herpes infection.

The next day, I admitted a second young woman with the same symptoms. She had also had intercourse with the same rock star on the same weekend.

Herpes is terribly infectious. Approximately one-third of unmarried sexually active people have contracted herpes by the age of thirty. Most people who develop herpes in the genital area will continue to have outbreaks for the rest of their lives. The first outbreak is called the primary infection and is the infection that hurts most severely. The outbreaks that occur after the first one are called secondary infections. Although they are usually much less painful than the primary one, they can be troubling as they revisit year after year.

It is not unusual to be infectious without knowing it. Everyone who has herpes outbreaks can spread the herpes virus between outbreaks because cells of the virus are intermittently shed or discarded by the body, even when an infection has subsided. People who know they have herpes often feel "safe" having sex if they do not at that moment have an outbreak.

Not only does the herpes virus shed a few hours before the actual outbreak and continue to shed for a while after the outbreak has subsided, but also herpes sores can be so small and painless that an outbreak is barely noticeable and therefore considered unimportant. In addition, apparently normal skin and vaginal lining in a herpes-infected individual can shed the virus even though there is no sore. A few people with herpes have never had a noticeable sore.

> Herpes is terribly infectious. Approximately one-third of unmarried sexually active people have contracted herpes by the age of thirty.

Although herpes is not especially dangerous unless it infects the eyes, the brain, or a baby (see below), it is painful, embarrassing, annoying, and expensive. It can interfere with intercourse. One of my patients was married to a man who had occasional herpes outbreaks that did not bother him much. She became infected and the infections bothered her almost continually. She had outbreaks several times each month and often could not have intercourse because of the pain. Her herpes was resistant to Zovirax. Eventually she and her husband divorced.

herpes in men

In men, the blisters and sores caused by the genital herpes virus may appear on the penis, scrotum, or anus. Herpes outbreaks in men are generally not as painful as in women but are still highly infectious.

herpes in women

In women, the blisters and sores caused by the genital herpes virus may appear on the vulva, inside the vagina, on the cervix, or in the anal region.

Sexually transmitted genital herpes poses a grave threat to newborn babies. If a woman delivers vaginally during her first outbreak of genital herpes, her baby has a 40 to 50 percent chance of becoming infected. If the baby becomes infected, it has a 60 percent chance of dying. Infected babies who survive have a 50 percent chance of being severely brain damaged. Herpes is a horrible infection for a baby and a terrifying infection for a pregnant woman because of the potential for infecting her baby.

If a woman has a recurrent herpes outbreak at the time she delivers, there is a 5 percent chance of the baby becoming infected—still a frightening prospect for the parents and the doctor. Even though this is a low percentage, doctors usually recommend that pregnant women who have a herpes outbreak at the time of delivery have a cesarean section.

diagnosing herpes

The invading herpes virus may be either *herpes simplex type I* or *type II.* Although years ago physicians thought type II always caused genital herpes and type I caused fever blisters, studies have clearly shown that either virus can cause genital herpes and either virus can cause fever blisters.

The herpes virus does not reside in the area where initial contact is made. It invades the body and makes its way up the nerves from the infected area, finally lodging in groups of nerve cells (ganglia) located near the spinal cord. When it causes its typical sores, the virus has to come back down the nerves to the genitals.

The first herpes outbreak is usually much more severe than later recurrences. It can cause enlarged lymph nodes in the groin. Flulike symptoms may occur in the form of fever and muscle aches.

The initial infection from an encounter with a partner who has herpes will occur within two to fourteen days. An experienced doctor may be able to tell by looking at a blister whether or not it is herpes. The doctor will swab the sore to obtain secretions to send to the laboratory. If the culture proves positive, herpes is present; if it is negative, the patient may or may not have herpes, since culture results can be inaccurate 15 to 20 percent of the time. A culture might be repeated if another outbreak occurs, but if the outbreak is in the same spot and appears typical of herpes, a culture is hardly necessary.

The herpes culture procedure is expensive. Somewhat less costly tests can be done, but they are less accurate. A blood test will indicate whether or not one has ever been infected with the herpes virus, but it is not useful in determining whether or not herpes has recently occurred.

The first sign of recurrent herpes outbreaks will usually be mild localized pain, tingling, itching, or burning. After the blisters form, they usually break open, leaving small, superficial sores that may vary from as small as an eighth of an inch to more than an inch across.

We are fairly certain now that most people who have been infected with herpes will develop these recurrent outbreaks periodically for many years, perhaps for life. New outbreaks may occur several times a month or only a few times a year. Women often find that their menstrual periods bring on a herpes episode. Intercourse, stress, and tight clothes often seem to cause recurrences. The outbreaks may be painful or almost unnoticeable—so minor that a person might not realize the small sore or insignificant bump is in fact a herpes lesion.

treating herpes

There is no medical cure for any virus, including herpes. Medication can reduce the troublesome aspects of herpes but cannot cure it. For an outbreak of herpes, whether fever blisters or genital sores, Zovirax ointment can be applied to the sores every three hours, or Zovirax pills or capsules can be taken. With this treatment the sores will usually be less painful and disappear more quickly than if left untreated. Generally the pills work more effectively than the ointment.

Two choices are now offered for preventing recurrent episodes of herpes. One can take Zovirax (or similar) pills every day, month after month. About 40 to 75 percent of herpes sufferers will have no recurrences while taking this daily medication. Another approach is to wait until the tingling of the skin develops just before a herpes outbreak and then immediately start taking Zovirax and continue taking it until all signs of herpes are gone. This will often prevent a sore from developing. Fortunately, Zovirax seems to be a safe drug.

Other drugs like Zovirax have been developed. Your doctor can tell you which drug is best for you.

long–term effects of herpes

Although herpes is inconvenient and uncomfortable, there is very little medical danger from the infection unless a person has an impaired immune system due to, for example, chemotherapy or AIDS. Herpes does not cause cancer and it almost never causes permanent injury unless it infects a person's eyes or brain or infects a newborn baby.

One of the worst aggravations of recurrent herpes is when it happens. Unfortunately, it has a way of surfacing at the most inconvenient, inappropriate times: on a vacation when wearing a tight swimsuit, during stressful times such as final exams, deadlines at work, preparations for a wedding ceremony. Outbreaks at such times can seem a true disaster.

The most severe and widespread effect of herpes is its emotional impact. An article, "Fever All Through the Night," by Nora Gallagher in *Mother Jones Magazine* (7:9, 1982) gives an accurate description of the emotional havoc herpes causes:

> If you listen to what herpes victims say, the overriding feelings they have are anger and guilt. Part of the anger is due to having an incurable disease in an age when almost anything can be fixed and, once fixed, forgotten. Guilt arises because it is currently fashionable to place some blame on the patient for getting sick. Add to that a disease that comes and goes of its own free will, and you have a feeling of helplessness.
>
> There is also the worry of being contagious. It is hard to convey how terrible some herpes sufferers feel about carrying around a disease. They feel, they say, like lepers. They feel "disgusting, sleasy" and the feelings are compounded if the person gives the virus to someone else.
>
> According to the Herpes Resource Center [herpes victims] are usually well-educated, middle- to upper-class. They are used to having a lot of control over their lives. They are used to being healthy. Herpes directly attacks their sense of control.
>
> Finally, there is the sexual guilt, perhaps the most pervasive of all herpes symptoms. "I felt I deserved it," said Linda, "because I picked it up while going through a promiscuous stage." This guilt is reinforced by the over-reactions of others. Linda's roommate used to scrub out the bathtub with Comet after Linda used it and before she herself stepped in.

preventing herpes

Herpes is such an aggravating problem that it is worth doing whatever it takes to avoid infection. Condoms may reduce the risk of infection provided they are used with every act of intercourse. A sex partner may be infectious even if no sore is present. As a matter of fact, most people become herpes infected when they have intercourse with someone who does not have a sore. Therefore, a partner's sexual secretions must be prevented from ever coming into contact with not only the sexual organs but also the skin of the vaginal area (or the mouth, if oral sex is practiced). One act of intercourse without a condom may give a person herpes.

Herpes is a *sexually* transmitted disease that is almost always contracted through intercourse or other intimate physical contact. The only way it can be caught from a toilet seat is by coming in direct contact with moist secretions that have very recently been left on the seat by someone else. It is almost never transmitted by shaking hands or hugging or similar contact with a victim.

Herpes, and all sexually transmitted diseases, cause increasing frustration and complications. How much better it is to avoid infection than to cope with it after becoming infected. If you are saving sex for marriage, relax, and do not worry about herpes. You will almost certainly not get it. Enjoy the freedom and safety that are yours.

7

syphilis

ABOUT 50% OF SYPHILIS PATIENTS ARE UNAWARE OF ITS PRESENCE OR CONSIDER LESIONS INCONSEQUENTIAL.

MORE THAN 50% OF WOMEN WHO HAVE INTERCOURSE ONE TIME WITH A MAN WHO HAS SYPHILIS WILL BECOME INFECTED.

SYPHILIS LESIONS INCREASE 9 TIMES THE DANGER OF BECOMING INFECTED WITH HIV.

THIS IS A TRUE STORY. I TELL IT BECAUSE I WANT TO CHALLENGE the false assumption that young people who attend a "good" high school or a prestigious major university are somehow immune from becoming infected with an STD such as syphilis.

A young university woman allowed a fellow student to talk her into having intercourse. A couple of weeks after that episode she developed a small, painless genital sore and went to the Student Health Center. A few cultures were done but they did not reveal the cause of her problem. So she saw one of my associates. He tested her and found she had syphilis, treated her with penicillin, and cured her.

She was fortunate. Many people ignore a syphilis sore because it is painless. However, after the initial sore heals, the infection goes underground in the body, to silently wreak its havoc. Most victims are then totally unaware of its presence. It is difficult to identify its nearly silent but relentless multiplication without a blood test.

Syphilis is an infection caused by a germ called a spirochete, so named because of its somewhat corkscrew appearance. The syphilis organism dies quickly if it is not in a warm, moist environment. It can be transmitted only from one moist area to another.

Syphilis infection begins at the moment of contact. The initial sore called a chancre (shanker) will appear within ten days to three months. The average time is three weeks after initial contact. Blood tests are not accurate until at least a week, maybe a month, after the lesion appears. While the most common mode of transmission is intercourse or genital contact, documented studies have indicated that infections have been transmitted by kissing. Any contact with broken skin is an open highway for the syphilis organism.

An infection with syphilis may increase by approximately nine times the possibility that a man or woman can be infected with HIV. Any ulcerative disease of the genitals can make the body much more susceptible to HIV infection.

While it is not against the law to have syphilis and your doctor will not report it to the police department, doctors are required to make a confidential report to the local public health department if a patient is found to have syphilis. This allows the health department to trace this silent killer and identify people who are unaware that they are infected and passing on the disease.

syphilis in women

A woman will usually develop a chancre during the initial stage of syphilis. Since it can be high inside her vagina, she might be unaware of its presence. This sore is almost always painless so a woman may have no clues that she has become infected. If she has engaged in oral sex, she may have a chancre on her lips that would be noticeable. A chancre on her vulva would also be noticeable.

If a woman becomes pregnant, she must have a blood test for syphilis, because syphilis can be severely damaging to a baby. If her sex partner has not been recently tested for syphilis and there is a possibility that he might be infected, he should also have a blood test and they should avoid sex until the results of the tests are known or until the baby is born.

syphilis in men

Usually a man will be more aware of the initial stage of syphilis than a woman because he would have a noticeable chancre on his penis, scrotum, or lips. Men need to remember that this chancre will be painless. Therefore, if a man has a genital sore, he should see a doctor even if the sore is not painful. Syphilis can be difficult to diagnose and it is important to tell your doctor if there is any possibility that you could be infected with an STD.

A man in the latent stage of syphilis is not as likely to transmit the disease to a sex partner as he is in the primary and secondary stages. A woman, however, can often transmit syphilis during the menstrual period, even in the latent phase.

The following paragraphs explain secondary and latent syphilis. Symptoms will be the same for both men and women.

diagnosing syphilis

When the initial episode of syphilis produces a chancre, your doctor may microscopically examine a smear of the secretions from the chancre. If it is syphilis, the spirochetes will usually be identifiable. If either of you suspect that you might have syphilis, you should be checked for any physical changes that are typical of a syphilitic infection. Even if you have no identifiable changes, you could still be infected, so a blood test for syphilis should be done. If you are the least bit worried about the possibility that you may have syphilis, have a syphilis blood test.

Syphilis sores may appear on the skin of the vulva, in the vagina (or on the penis), in the mouth, or on the lips. It is common for a woman to have more than one chancre with a first syphilis infection.

A chancre often starts as an ulcer but later becomes a knot, with a punched-out, thickened base and firm, rolled edges. Some chancres may remain soft. Because there is no pain, many people ignore these seemingly insignificant sores and do not see a doctor.

Secondary syphilis develops six weeks to six months after the initial infection. This second stage is when the disease is most infectious. Symptoms may include headache, fatigue, low-grade fever, skin rash, and enlarged lymph nodes.

Condyloma lata (raised growths, which are flat-topped, moist, and gray in color) may develop in this stage. The growths may become ulcerated and thickened and ooze some fluid. These condyloma, which may appear in the mouth, beneath the breasts, and under the arms, teem with spirochetes, and are extremely infectious. Enlargement of the lymph nodes in the groin usually accompanies the appearance of *condyloma lata*.

> When syphilis reaches the late stage, devastating, irreversible medical problems may emerge in almost any part of the body.

Secondary syphilis will pass, even without treatment. At that time the signs of syphilis will disappear spontaneously, and a latent period will follow, lasting from several months to twenty years. During the latent period, there are no outward symptoms of syphilis and the disease is relatively contained. It is still quietly destroying portions of the body's tissues during this time, however. Entire organs of the body can be destroyed.

When syphilis reaches the late stage, devastating, irreversible medical problems may emerge in almost any part of the body. Some of the more common effects are aneurysms of the cardiovascular system, deterioration of the central nervous system, damage to bones, and damage to peripheral nerves.

treating syphilis

The standard treatment for syphilis is penicillin, a drug that continues to be 100 percent effective in killing the organism that causes the disease. Alternative antibiotics are available for those allergic to penicillin.

long–term effects of syphilis

If syphilis is not diagnosed and treated, it will silently destroy the victim's body day after day and year after year. Then, when the disease is recognized and the infection is treated, much damage may have already been done. The effects of syphilis will usually not get worse once the spirochetes are killed, but getting rid of the germs will not reverse the damage already done.

One major threat that occurs during all stages of syphilis is damage to the unborn child of a syphilitic mother. Congenital syphilis is often a disaster. About 20 percent of pregnancies complicated by syphilis end in miscarriages or stillbirths. Within the first month, 15 percent of babies born to a syphilitic mother will die. Of those who survive, one-third will have some permanent abnormality, such as obstruction of the nasal passages, flattening of the bridge of the nose, fractures of the bones, enlarged liver and spleen, or eye and ear damage.

8

hepatitis B

IN THE U.S. AT LEAST 100,000 PEOPLE ANNUALLY ARE INFECTED WITH HEPATITIS B AS A RESULT OF SEXUAL INTERCOURSE.

HEPATITIS B IS 10 TIMES MORE INFECTIOUS THAN HIV.

ABOUT 60 TO 70% OF SEXUALLY ACTIVE MALE HOMOSEXUALS HAVE A HEPATITIS B INFECTION.

HEPATITIS B IS THE MOST COMMON CAUSE OF LIVER CANCER IN THE U.S.; BETWEEN 5,000 AND 6,000 AMERICANS DIE FROM LIVER CANCER OR CIRRHOSIS EACH YEAR.

TWENTY YEARS AGO HEPATITIS B WAS FIRST DISCOVERED TO be sexually transmitted and now it is known to be one of the most common STDs in the world. Hepatitis B is an extremely infectious virus transmitted in sexual secretions, saliva, and blood. Male homosexual activity is unusually effective in transmitting hepatitis B, being three to twenty times more likely to infect people than heterosexual sex. As with AIDS, there are other ways to transmit the disease. Blood transfusions, getting infected blood on a break in the skin, or using contaminated intravenous needles can cause a hepatitis B infection.

Three young high school men in our area developed hepatitis B about a year after graduation. All three had had intercourse with the same woman just before graduation. Tracking by the health department revealed the woman had had intercourse with five other men during the same period of time. Two were located and found to be uninfected. Three men could not be located. The possibility exists that they are now infected with hepatitis B and are passing it on to unsuspecting partners.

This scenario is being repeated across the U.S. It is possible to have hepatitis B and not be aware of the infection. That ignorance will not prevent a person from passing on the virus to a sex partner.

Not only can a person have hepatitis B without being aware of it, but he or she can also be a chronic carrier of the disease for years without knowing it. Carriers may presently feel no ill effects (or have already recovered from them), but for the rest of their lives they might infect those with whom they have sex.

A study of university students conducted in 1986 confirmed that a person who has had fewer than ten sex partners has a relatively low risk of getting hepatitis B. That relatively low risk factor is not much comfort to those three young men described above. Those who have had more than ten sex partners are at a much greater risk of being infected with hepatitis B.

> There is no known cure for hepatitis B.

hepatitis B in men and women

Typically, a person infected with hepatitis B initially develops jaundice (yellowing of the skin and whites of the eyes), tiredness, nausea, dark urine, and gray-colored stools. This clears up after a few weeks. The infected person, however, may still have the virus in his or her liver, causing chronic infection, an occurrence in about 10 percent of hepatitis B patients. The chronic infection can result in cancer of the liver or cirrhosis, both of which can ultimately lead to the need for a liver transplant or result in death.

Persons who become chronic carriers can, for the rest of their lives, pass the disease along to any sex partner, health-care professional, or anyone who comes into contact with bodily secretions or blood.

An infected pregnant woman can transmit hepatitis B to her baby, possibly making the child a carrier for life. Even worse, 40 to 50 percent of these children who do become carriers will develop cancer of the liver. Others may develop severe liver disease such as cirrhosis. Most obstetricians order a routine test for hepatitis B on all pregnant women. If a mother has the disease a baby should receive immunoglobulin at birth, followed by a series of vaccine injections to prevent him or her from becoming infected with this virus.

diagnosing hepatitis B

A blood test would be ordered if a person has the typical symptoms of hepatitis (see paragraphs above). However, sometimes the disease produces few or no symptoms. After the initial infection is over and all symptoms have disappeared, the blood test will remain positive for hepatitis B. The blood tests also reveal whether or not a person has become a carrier of hepatitis B. Those who are carriers of hepatitis B can infect others for the rest of their lives.

treating hepatitis B

There is no known cure for hepatitis B. As with other forms of hepatitis, the treatment for hepatitis B is nonspecific supportive care which includes rest as a primary part of the regimen. Most people recover from the infection but some become carriers and have the infection without symptoms for years.

Anyone who suspects exposure to the hepatitis B virus should immediately contact a doctor's office since immunoglobulin may provide some protection, if given promptly.

9

HIV/AIDS

AIDS IS NOW THE LEADING CAUSE OF DEATH IN AMERICANS AGES 25–44.

APPROXIMATELY 7,000 HIV INFECTED MOTHERS ARE DELIVERING BABIES EACH YEAR. BETWEEN 1,000 AND 2,000 OF THE BABIES WILL HAVE HIV. PRACTICALLY ALL OF THE MOTHERS WILL DIE OF AIDS.

ABOUT 25% OF NEWLY DIAGNOSED HIV PATIENTS ARE BELOW AGE 22.

HIV IS A MINDLESS GERM. IT DOES NOT CHOOSE A VICTIM TO infect; it merely tags along with blood or sexual secretions. The only way to avoid this menacing virus is to avoid contact with another person's blood or sexual secretions. If a person decides to save sex for marriage, then there is little need to worry about HIV unless the marriage partner has HIV.

At our local high school I shared the lecture platform with Sherry Root, an AIDS victim. I talked about the risks of having and reasons for avoiding premarital sex. The teenagers listened attentively. But when Sherry told her story, the best illustration of the devastation of sexually transmitted disease and HIV that I had heard, the audience was spellbound. This is Sherry's story as it was reported in the *Austin American Statesman,* Tuesday, December 8, 1992.

> She grew up in a middle-class family in northwest Austin. She didn't drink, she didn't smoke, she didn't do drugs. While

in college, she began dating a guy she met at school who was from a small town outside Austin. She was nineteen at the time, and they dated for two years. It was her first sexual relationship, and Root says they discussed birth-control methods and decided she should take the pill.

It was not until four years later, engaged to be married, and on a vacation with her fiance, that Root began to suspect that something was wrong. She was fatigued, running a fever, and would wake up nights soaked in sweat. She also had lost quite a bit of weight and began having problems catching her breath.

She went to see a doctor. He told her it was viral pneumonia and gave her medicine. But three weeks later she was no better. In fact, she was much worse. She could not get out of bed, couldn't even roll over without help. Her father had to carry her into the doctor's office because she was too weak to walk. She took an HIV test that day.

"I knew it was going to be negative. I was confident it would be negative because things like that didn't happen to people like me. I was a good girl. I didn't date people with sexually transmitted diseases."

Then on July 30, 1991, a day that would be etched in her memory, Root learned that she had AIDS. She discovered later that her first boyfriend, who had experimented with intravenous drugs as a teenager, had known for more than three years that he had AIDS and had not told her. He died in March 1992.

Sherry asked, "What is it that I can say that can convince you that you are at risk? I come here not because I have to but because I care. I come here because I hope you are never in the position I am in today. I come here today to leave little pieces of myself with you so that maybe some little thing I have said will stick in your mind and make you think before you act the next time.

"I'll never be able to get married, never be able to have children, never be able to give my parents grandchildren, never be able to grow old and get gray hair—all because of a choice I made when I was nineteen."

Since that time Sherry Root died of a disease she never in her wildest imagination dreamed she would contract.

I plead with you, do not let this happen to you. HIV is a relentless, terrible, frightening, immediate threat to anyone who has sex outside of a lifelong, monogamous relationship with an uninfected person.

> HIV tags along with blood or sexual secretions. It is an almost perfect killing machine.

Since so many sexually active singles in our society are infected with STDs, they serve as a fertile field for HIV infection to occur. If you have chlamydia, gonorrhea, or bacterial vaginosis, you are three to five times more more likely to get HIV if you have sex with someone who is HIV infected. If you have another STD, one like herpes that causes ulcers, you are approximately nine times more likely to be infected with HIV when you have sex with a person who is HIV infected. Just because you already have one STD does not mean you will be immune to another STD. Chances are actually greater that you will become infected.

HIV/AIDS in men and women

A word of warning: Don't let these paragraphs of information about AIDS which sound so mechanical or medical lull you into a sense of complacency. Do not allow these facts to mask the human devastation that Sherry Root and other AIDS victims experienced. AIDS is a horrendous, heart-wrenching disease.

Acquired Immune Deficiency Syndrome (AIDS) is a viral infection caused by the human immunodeficiency virus (HIV). This retrovirus selectively attacks the immune cells in the human body. However, brain and spinal cord cells can also be damaged. Some experts have described it as an almost perfect killing machine.

Once an HIV infection occurs, it spreads to all the cells of the immune system, destroying them as it goes. The human immunodeficiency virus mutates more than most other known human viruses. Over 150 strains of HIV have already been identified.

When persons become HIV infected, they are said to be HIV positive. Infection usually occurs from sexual activity, using contaminated needles for intravenous injection of street drugs, or HIV contaminated blood transfusions. It is not spread by mosquitoes, hand contact, or hugging. You can become infected with HIV from only one sexual encounter with an HIV infected sex partner. If you become infected with HIV, you will be contagious from the time of the initial infection, even before a blood test is positive.

The first symptoms of HIV infection are often flulike: aching all over, fever, enlarged lymph nodes. These symptoms soon pass and the victim feels restored to health. From that point on, this person is HIV infected and will be HIV positive for his or her lifetime. If sexual secretions or blood is given to another person, that person can become infected with HIV. During this latent period, the HIV has gone underground and the HIV victim will not know he or she has the disease unless testing is done.

This latent, or silent, period can last for up to ten years, or maybe longer. When the immune system has been so severely damaged that the body cannot defend itself against infections, the person begins having pneumonia and other problems, such as those Sherry experienced.

A common complaint is enlarged lymph nodes, especially in the back of the neck and under the arms, as the body attempts to fight off infections that normally would not be a threat. Other symptoms are intermittent fever, weight loss, persistent diarrhea, painful candida (fungus) mouth infections, and shingles.

When these health problems surface, the person is said to have AIDS. The presence of AIDS can be confirmed by a blood test. If a blood test reveals fewer than 200 CD4+ lymphocytes per microliter, an HIV positive person has progressed to AIDS. These CD4+ lymphocytes are the immune cells that circulate in the bloodstream and fight infection. Once an immune system is severely deficient, three major types of problems commonly develop. These are called "opportunistic" infections, infections that would not normally infect a healthy person. These include pneumocystis carinii pneumonia, toxoplasmosis, and cytomegalovirus infections. Other possible AIDS related problems that could develop are non-Hodgkin's lymphoma and Kaposi's sarcoma. AIDS encephalitis, with dementia, is another possibility. Within a year of the development of any of these AIDS symptoms, 50 percent of the victims die. About 90 percent of AIDS victims with these symptoms die within three years. One thing is clear: there are no AIDS survivors.

A few people are HIV infected but do not develop the antibodies necessary to produce a positive HIV blood test. There is absolutely no way for these people or anyone else to know they have HIV, yet they are infectious to other people. When they finally develop AIDS, their HIV condition can be confirmed by a blood test. This is a rare condition, but keep this in mind if you are planning to have sex with someone who has had sex with several partners or has other potential risk factors for HIV infection.

If you do have a new sex partner, be checked not only for HIV but also for syphilis and hepatitis B after six months. Even if you have had sex with that person only one time, I recommend that you have these tests. Additionally, you should be checked for chlamydia and gonorrhea within a month after you have a new sex partner. Do not have sex with anyone until they have had all five of these tests, no matter how normal and healthy they look.

There is a way to be totally safe from all of these diseases: have sex with only one person and be sure that person is having sex only with you. If the two of you stay together for the rest of your lives, neither one ever has to worry about any STD.

diagnosing HIV/AIDS

The blood tests now done for HIV look for the body's reaction to HIV. When the body becomes infected with HIV, it develops antibodies to try to fight off the disease. The HIV blood test looks for those antibodies. It takes a few months to develop antibodies. Any blood test taken immediately after contracting HIV would be negative. A blood test would not be positive until the antibodies could be detected. Within three months, 95 percent of people with HIV will have a positive blood test; within six months, almost all of them will have a positive blood test.

The ELISA (enzyme-linked immunosorbent assay) blood test is presently the best screening test for HIV. If the ELISA test is positive twice, a Western Blot test is done to confirm the accuracy of the ELISA.

A new antigen test will probably have been released by the FDA by the time this book is printed. This test detects the virus itself; it actually finds the HIV organism. It can be used to find HIV even when the body has not yet developed antibodies. Blood banks will be mandated to use this test on all their blood products.

treating HIV/AIDS

There is no known cure for AIDS. All HIV infected individuals will probably develop AIDS and eventually die from its effects.

AZT (zidovudine) is a drug that helps suppress viral activity but it is not a cure. Other drugs are used to treat AIDS, but they only help to control complications.

Researchers are pessimistic about the prospects of finding either a cure for AIDS or a vaccine to prevent it. Scientists seem unable to find a cure for any virus infection, let alone a stubborn one like AIDS.

AIDS victims usually take the medications and do the procedures that can help prolong life and make it more comfortable. This requires that they take multiple medications either as pills or shots. They may need to have a tube permanently placed into one of their veins for the injection of drugs directly into the bloodstream. Other uncomfortable and painful procedures may need to be tolerated. But all of these things are merely postponement of the inevitable. The death that occurs with AIDS is not an easy death—and it will always come.

Obvious dangers of AIDS are increasing debilitation and death. Another, not so well-known, danger affects the 7,000 children born to HIV infected mothers each year. If the mother receives AZT while she is pregnant only about 8 percent of those babies are born infected. About 25 percent of babies born to mothers who do not receive treatment for HIV are born infected or contract the infection through breast feeding. Sadly, in addition to the fact that all infected babies will die, so will practically all HIV infected mothers, leaving their noninfected babies motherless.

condoms and HIV/AIDS

Contrary to what you may have been taught, condoms do not offer reliable protection against HIV infection. One study used to prove that condoms are reliable for HIV prevention did not involve a large enough group of patients to reliably prove the protective benefits of condom use. Only 124 patients in the study used condoms consistently and correctly.

A much more helpful study is one done by Dr. Susan Weller at the University of Texas in 1993. She looked at the results of ten studies on the effectiveness of condoms in preventing HIV transmission from an infected person to an uninfected person. She found **an average failure rate of 31 percent**. Almost one out of three times the condom allowed HIV transmission from an infected person to an uninfected person. Dr. Weller concludes: "It is a disservice to encourage the belief that condoms will prevent the spread of HIV."

Most of these studies ran for only two years. If they had been extended for a longer period, the failure rates may have been even higher. Condoms, at best, do not eliminate the risk of getting HIV; they only minimize it.

10

sexually transmitted vaginal infections

ORGANISMS THAT CAUSE PESKY VAGINAL INFECTIONS ARE USUALLY NOT TROUBLESOME FOR MEN.

BACTERIAL VAGINOSIS SIGNIFICANTLY INCREASES THE RISK OF HAVING A PREMATURE DELIVERY.

ALTHOUGH SEXUALLY TRANSMITTED VAGINAL INFECTIONS ARE common, a woman who is a virgin until marriage and then stays married to a man who has never had intercourse with another person will probably have only one type of vaginal infection. She may have candida, also called fungus, yeast, or monilia infection. Usually this infection is eliminated with the use of Monistat, GyneLotrimin, or some other medication. Some women, especially diabetics, seem prone to recurring fungus infections. Usually these infections do not produce significant emotional consequences.

Much different and more serious are the vaginal infections of a woman who has had more than one sex partner or has sex with a man who has had other sex partners. The multiple exposures that occur when people have intercourse with more than one person can cause persistent, bothersome, odorous infections that can be difficult to eliminate.

Although men who have contracted these infections occasionally may have a discharge from the penis or slight burn-

> The multiple exposures that occur when people have intercourse with more than one person can cause persistent, bothersome, odorous infections that can be difficult to eliminate.

ing with urination, they usually have no symptoms. Infected men are usually not aware that they are carrying or passing on these germs.

One of my patients had a stubborn vaginal infection. I prescribed oral antibiotics and antibiotic creams, changing medications in an effort to find one that would eliminate the infection. Finally we were successful. She changed sex partners the next year and came back with a similar infection. Again extensive, expensive treatment was required to clear the second infection.

Some gynecologists refer to this problem as "dirty vagina"–not a flattering term. When a woman has intercourse with a man who has had intercourse with other women, he ejaculates into her not only sperm and mucus but also all the germs he is carrying from other women. These germs can start growing in the vagina and produce discharge, odor, and discomfort. Women often become extremely frustrated by the discomfort, inconvenience, expense, and length of treatment required to eliminate a vaginal infection.

A couple of these organisms may cause some long-term effects in a woman's body. Trichomoniasis has some significant relationship to fallopian tube damage and resulting infertility. This relationship has not been absolutely proven but evidence currently available seems to indicate that the more episodes of trichomoniasis a woman has, the more likely she is to have obstructed fallopian tubes.

Even worse is new information about bacterial vaginosis, an infection usually sexually transmitted. Physicians label this as BV and researchers have found that this infection significantly increases a woman's risk of having a premature delivery. About 10 percent of childbearing women have this infection. In some areas as many as 33 percent are infected.

Using condoms is not a reliable, effective way to avoid sexually transmitted vaginal infections. The diseased organisms are thoroughly mixed into a man's sexual secretions and even the slightest bit that is spilled may be enough to cause an infection in the woman.

trichomoniasis

Trichomonal vaginitis causes a vaginal discharge and itching of the vulva. The itching can be quite intolerable, bothersome enough to send a woman to her physician. Tenderness and burning of the vulva frequently accompany the infection, leading to pain with intercourse.

Trichomoniasis is now one of the most common sexually transmitted diseases in the world. About 90 percent of prostitutes have this infection at one time or another.

Although men who have contracted this infection occasionally have a discharge from the penis or slight burning with urination, they usually have no symptoms.

bacterial vaginosis

Almost invariably sexually transmitted, this infection is caused by the germ *Gardnerella vaginalis* mixed with other germs. A woman with BV will have a vaginal discharge that may initially be misinterpreted as only normal vaginal secretions. Aside from the messy discharge, there often is an accompanying fishy odor. The vulvar area may have mild burning and itching.

Infected men usually have no symptoms of BV and can unknowingly pass it on to their sex partners.

diagnosing vaginitis

An examining doctor may notice that the patient has a watery vaginal discharge that itches, or the discharge may be frothy and slightly green. Under the microscope, the trichomonas protozoa may be seen moving around.

If the examining doctor notices that the patient has a vaginal discharge accompanied by odor and the secretions are slightly creamy and gray-colored, microsopic examination may reveal "clue cells." These are normal vaginal cells that have the *Gardnerella* organism stuck to them. Hundreds of small knots seem to be growing out of the vaginal cells. The knots are the BV germs.

Because a woman can be infected with either of these organisms and not have any symptoms, I recommend that a woman be tested for these germs every time she has a new sex partner or every time her sex partner has a new sex partner. These organisms can cause major problems and there is no other way for a woman to protect herself from the potential damage of these infections without knowing she has the infection and seeking treatment to eliminate it.

treating trichomonas
and bacterial vaginosis

The only treatment for trichomonas vaginitis is Flagyl (metronidazole). It can be prescribed in pill or cream form, or as an injectible medication. Repeated doses may be needed if the infection is tenacious and resists treatments. The sex partner of a woman with trichomonas must also be treated to prevent reinfecting her. It is recommended that sexual intercourse be avoided until the treatment period is completed. Some trichomonas organisms are becoming resistant to metronidazole. This is a concern for both patients and physicians because there is no other effective drug for trichomonas.

Flagyl vaginal cream (Metro-Gel Vaginal) is an effective treatment for BV. Clindamycin (Cleocin), an antibiotic vaginal cream, also seems to be effective against BV. Since BV is usually sexually transmitted it is important that the sex partner of a woman who is being treated with vaginal cream receive oral treatment with Flagyl pills.

long – term effects of vaginitis

I have already pointed out that trichomonas may cause tubal damage with possible infertility and that bacterial vaginosis can cause premature labor.

Startling information about these diseases has recently been released. A woman who has bacterial vaginosis is significantly more likely to become infected with HIV if she has intercourse with an HIV infected partner.

It is common for a person who is infected with one STD to also have a second or third one. So it is extremely important to be tested for other STDs if BV or trichomonas infection is already present.

For your own peace of mind, and for your health, have intercourse with no one until you are married. Marry someone who has also held to these standards and both of you will avoid the nightmares and heartaches of STDs. If you marry someone who had a sex partner in the past and you develop trichomonas or BV, get treatment immediately. If you never again change sex partners, you should be free from worry once the infection is cured.

11

other sexually transmitted diseases

INFECTION WITH A "MINOR" STD DOES NOT MAKE ONE IM-
MUNE TO A "MAJOR" ONE.

ANY STD INFECTION CAN BE EMOTIONALLY AND PHYSICALLY
DEVASTATING.

ONE OF MY PATIENTS DID NOT CONSIDER HERSELF PROMISCU-
ous. She changed sex partners "only once in a while." Although I had warned her repeatedly about the probability
of acquiring an STD if she continued her lifestyle, she dismissed my warnings as overly cautious and unnecessary.

So when she came in for her annual checkup, she dismissed
the persistent itching in her pubic hair as being an allergic
reaction to bubble bath or detergent. She had pubic lice. I
found the characteristic "nits" or eggs that the lice lay on
pubic hair. She was amazed and embarrassed.

Actually she was fortunate. The man who gave her lice
could also have given her a much more dangerous STD.
Pubic lice are often present in people who have had multiple sex partners and who have poor hygiene.

There are many other sexually transmitted diseases which
are relatively infrequent or uncomplicated. Be aware though
that any infection with an STD can be emotionally and physically devastating, even if it is considered a "minor" STD.

Remember that an infection with a "minor" STD will not make you immune to infection from a "major," potentially deadly STD.

nonspecific urethritis and prostatitis

Two problems of the male genitals are caused by STD. These are nonspecific urethritis and prostatitis.

Nonspecific urethritis means a urethral infection from an STD organism, usually chlamydia or gonorrhea. Generally it results in a mild burning on urination and a urethral discharge with a slight amount of pus. If a man has a gonorrhea infection, his penile discharge may be heavy. If he has a chlamydia infection, the discharge may be mild with almost no burning with urination. Either one of these problems needs to be treated promptly. An infection from gonorrhea can result in scarring that is so severe a man cannot urinate or ejaculate. Major surgery may be required to rebuild a tube for urination and ejaculation. A chlamydia infection merely causes a mild discharge but a man may pass this infection on to a woman. If she gets chlamydia, she can become sterile from pelvic inflammatory disease.

Prostatitis from STD would be comparable to vaginitis. Chlamydia can cause vaginal discharge in a woman and prostatitis in a man. Other STD organisms can also cause prostatitis, which for a man can be even more of a problem than vaginitis for a woman. Prostatitis is a deepseated infection and can be difficult to cure. It often involves months of antibiotics and multiple visits to a physician.

pubic lice (crabs)

Commonly known a "crabs," pubic lice are visible to the naked eye. These tiny but bothersome creatures cause intense itching and irritation of the pubic skin. The inevitable scratching causes small sores that ooze pus. Most commonly passed from contact with pubic hair of an infected person, these organisms can also be transmitted by contact with infected clothing or bed sheets.

Pediculosis is the medical term used for lice infestation. Pubic lice do not infect the hair of the head and head lice do not infect pubic hair. There is no real consequence from lice except that they can be spread sexually and are quite irritating when present. Effective treatment is readily available. Medicated shampoo to kill the parasite is most often used. Bedclothes, towels, and undergarments must be washed thoroughly in hot water so reinfestation will not occur. The major danger is that the sex partner who has lice and spreads them can also be infected with a more dangerous STD.

Molluscum contagiosum

Before 1977 *Molluscum contagiosum* was not regarded as an STD. This condition is surprisingly common. In my practice I have seen *Molluscum contagiosum* more often than gonorrhea or syphilis. It is not a dangerous infection. People are startled and amazed when I diagnose wartlike growths on their inner thighs as an STD.

Skin-colored, slightly raised, and somewhat waxy-looking bumps are produced by this infection. The lesions have a slight indention in the center, and may occur singly or in groups. They are produced by a mildly contagious poxvirus and they are limited to skin irritation. The usual size of a lesion is about an eighth of an inch across. Sometimes the bumps protrude from the skin like a small tick. Growths may not appear for several weeks or months. They develop as bumps on the surface of the lower abdomen, the pubic area, the inner thighs, or the external genitalia. They may itch slightly but they do not hurt. There may be only one or several and they may be mistaken for ordinary pimples.

Usually the bumps do not clear up spontaneously, although they may. Treatment involves scraping out the small hard white core of each lesion. If the growths recur, the doctor may use cautery or trichloracetic acid after scraping them.

Both you and your sex partner can have *Molluscum contagiosum* without initially being aware of it. If you do have this infection, you should also be checked for other STDs as should your sex partner. If a person has one STD, it is possible to have others.

scabies

An intensely irritating infection, scabies is limited to the skin and victims most often seek out a dermatologist for treatment. Scabies is caused by a mite *(Sarcopetes scabiei),* a parasite of the skin. The mite burrows into the skin and forms a small, tortuous channel just under the surface. Its path can be seen with a magnifying glass. Favorite spots for the mites to burrow into are skin folds, the penis, scrotum, finger webs, wrists, elbows, nipples, umbilicus, buttocks, and insteps.

Scabies is transmitted from one person to another by skin-to-skin contact. Transmission is not necessarily sexual and can occur from bedclothes or undergarments only if they have been contaminated immediately beforehand. You can have scabies and not be aware that it was spread by close contact, possibly sexual. A person who showers regularly and stays clean may have itching in only a small area and not realize the cause of the problem.

Although not dangerous, scabies is bothersome. If the skin becomes badly irritated from scratching, impetigo (a bacterial infection) can develop. This secondary infection, if neglected, can lead to glomerulonephritis, a kidney disease.

The infection is diagnosed by looking at the area of itching with a magnifying instrument and discovering the burrowing channels. A superficial scrape of the skin of the burrow may help the doctor see the parasite itself. Treatment consists of applying a specific drug, such as Lindane, to all areas of the body, except the head. After eight hours, the body should be thoroughly washed and fresh clothing put on. The treatment is not recommended for pregnant women or lactating mothers. Anyone who has had close bodily contact with infected individuals, their clothing, or bed clothing, should receive treatment with Lindane or a similar drug.

chancroid, lymphogranuloma venereum (lgv), and granuloma inguinale (gi)

Each one of these diseases is caused by a different organism. The diseases are most commonly seen in warm tropical and subtropical climates and in populations with low standards of hygiene. All three are highly dangerous and destructive, causing the loss of vital tissue in the reproductive organs, gross enlargement of the sex organs, stricture of the intestines and rectum, obstruction of the anus, and even death.

The symptoms are quite apparent: tender lesions breaking down into painful ulcers, spreading over the genital area or skin surface of the stomach, groin, and thighs; bumps turning into raw, oozing masses of tissue and slow-healing lesions; a lesion with inflammatory swelling in the groin and accompanying fever, aches, and joint pains.

Both chancroid and granuloma inguinale (GI) produce sores and ulcers of the genital area. Anyone who has these symptoms will certainly be aware of them. Lymphogranuloma venereum (LGV) causes infection primarily of the colon. A person would not necessarily suspect an STD with the symptoms of diarrhea with blood and pus from the rectum. Fortunately these diseases generally respond quite well to antibiotics. If too much tissue has been destroyed because of delay in seeking treatment, however, resultant scarring can cause lingering medical problems.

Chancroid is much more common than LGV and GI. In the past, cultures for the organism that causes it were difficult to do and the results were not reliable. Now by testing for the DNA of *Haemophilus ducreyi,* the organism that causes chancroid, many more people are being diagnosed with it. All these diseases are risk factors for infection with HIV. Anyone with an ulcer in the genital area is more likely to become HIV infected.

other diseases that can be spread sexually

There are a number of infections that may or may not be sexually contracted but can be sexually transmitted. A pesky vaginal Candida (yeast) infection in a woman can be passed to her sex partner where it causes itching and irritation to the penis. The Epstein-Barr virus that can cause chronic illness has just recently been shown to be spread sexually. Shigella and salmonella bacterial infections which cause severe diarrhea can also be passed sexually.

cytomegalovirus infections (CMV)

A virus from the herpes group causes this disease. It can be passed by blood transfusions, intimate contact, and sexual intercourse. The disease is common in homosexual men and is also prevalent in men and women who have multiple sex partners. Newborns can be dangerously infected by the mother.

amebiasis

This parasitic infection, although not considered an STD, can be transmitted this way. It causes diarrhea and other intestinal problems. Complications may involve the liver. The infection is much more common in tropical regions than in the U.S.

giardiasis

Like amebiasis, this parasitic infection can cause diarrhea and, while not specifically an STD, it can definitely be passed sexually.

group A beta hemolytic streptococcal infection

While not considered an STD, this infection can be passed sexually. The germ is common and has been found in as many as 20 percent of all women. Rarely dangerous for the man or woman who becomes infected, it is devastating to newborns who become infected during labor and delivery.

mycoplasma infections

These common infections can be found in 7 to 20 percent of all people. While they do not harm men, in women they are associated with infertility and spontaneous abortion.

PART TWO

sexual fulfillment

behaviors and risks

12

mutual masturbation, outercourse, dry sex

STDS CAN BE TRANSMITTED WHETHER OR NOT VAGINAL IN-
TERCOURSE HAS OCCURRED.

STD ORGANISMS ARE USUALLY PRESENT IN A WOMAN'S
SECRETIONS.

EVEN A SMALL CRACK OR CUT OR A SKIN RASH CAN BE AN
ENTRYWAY FOR AN STD.

LIFE OFTEN PRESENTS US WITH CHOICES. WE MUST CHOOSE
one behavior or the other. The activities discussed in this
chapter involve behavior, and the choice you make will
affect your future life. One choice is to believe that emotional intimacy does not require physical or sexual contact. The other choice is to believe that participation in mutual masturbation, outercourse, and dry sex is not only
permissible, but even a healthy and important aspect of
one's sexuality.

What are these activities? *Dorland Medical Dictionary,*
28th ed, 1994, states that masturbation is "self-stimulation
of the genitals for sexual pleasure." *Mutual masturbation* is
a term used to refer to stimulation of another person's genital organs for sexual pleasure. Outercourse is genital contact without penetrative sex, either oral, anal, or vaginal.
The slang term *dry sex* is often used with reference to this
activity.

Many otherwise well-meaning people recommend that single persons engage in these activities. Are these activities potentially dangerous? Are they medically acceptable, safe alternatives to vaginal or oral sex? Are these ways to stay a virgin or to avoid sexually transmitted disease or pregancy and still engage in sexual activity? Good questions. One answer is the heartbreak of a young patient who listened to this message and tried it.

A thirteen-year-old patient adamantly maintained that she never had sex. On exam, she appeared to be a virgin but her vulvar skin biopsy showed precancer that had almost advanced to invasive cancer. She reported that she had participated in outercourse with her boyfriend.

She needed laser surgery treatment on her vulva. A follow-up exam about nine months later revealed she had carcinoma in situ of the vulva, which is an even closer step to cancer of the vulva. Removal of vulvar skin was necessary. Skin was grafted from her buttocks. Asthetically, her vulva is changed forever and will never appear normal.

Those who have never engaged in sexual activity need to know that it is "messy." Many people who experience their first encounter with sex are surprised at the messiness. The culmination of sexual activity for a man is ejaculation of a teaspoonful of semen: a wet, sticky fluid. Women experience vaginal lubrication which begins ten to thirty seconds after the onset of sexual stimulation (physical, psychological, or a combination of the two).

A woman masturbating a man will have her hands covered with his semen when he ejaculates. The hands of a man masturbating a woman will become quite moist from her vaginal secretions. Partners masturbating each other quite likely will touch their own genitals during the activity. Transmission

> Recent research has proven that STD organisms are present in and can be transmitted by sexual secretions.

of STDs may happen whether or not vaginal intercourse has occurred.

One study involved collection of semen specimens from men attending a clinic for treatment of genital warts. Some of the men in the study had warts just inside the urethra. In this location it would be impossible for the man or his partner to know he had warts. All the semen collected from these men revealed the presence of HPV organisms. About 95 percent of the men with warts in the uretha also had a second STD organism present. Any part of a woman's body that comes into contact (unknowingly!) with this infected semen can become infected, even if intercourse has not occurred. (This study was reported in *Genitourinary Medicine,* 1991.)

Another study reported that many (43 percent) HIV positive men have the virus in their pre-ejaculatory fluid. When men are sexually excited, they will often pass a small amount of secretion (pre-ejaculatory fluid) from the penis. When this fluid gets into even a tiny break in the skin of a sex partner, an STD infection can result. (This study was reported in *The Lancet* in December 1992.)

Chlamydia can be present in semen, but it can be difficult to find. A study conducted in 1993 involved semen donors who had already tested negative for chlamydia and were assumed to be acceptable for semen donations to fertility clinics. When DNA testing for chlamydia was performed on the semen donations, 10 percent tested positively for chlamydia and could infect women inseminated with their sperm. (This study was reported in *Fertility and Sterility,* 1993).

Do women's secretions carry STD organisms? A study of sexually active coeds at the University of California at Berkeley revealed that 46 percent had HPV infections (Bauer et al., *Journal of the American Medical Association,* 1991). The test involved a simple swabbing of the vagina.

A 1994 study involved secretions from the vagina and cervix of women without visible herpes who were in labor. Nine out of a hundred such women had the herpes virus present. (This study was reported in the *Journal of the American Medical Association*.)

If a woman has an STD, the organisms that cause disease will usually be present in her secretions. These diseases can be transmitted to a man who comes in contact with these secretions, even if penetrative intercourse does not occur.

Can pregnancy occur without vaginal sex? YES.

Sperm have the capacity to swim up the vaginal canal, through the cervix, and into the uterus. Sperm can do this whether they are deposited at the vaginal entrance or high inside the vagina. If semen is deposited at the woman's vaginal entrance, she does run the risk of becoming pregnant. Outercourse (dry sex) which involves close genital contact can cause pregnancy, even though the woman may technically still be a virgin.

Even though the medical data is clear that these are potentially dangerous practices, some otherwise reliable organizations recommend that early adolescents (ages 12–15) be taught that masturbation, alone or with a partner, is acceptable sexual behavior, that is, there is no risk of an STD or pregnancy from these activities.

For older students (ages 15–19), organizations such as the Sexuality Information and Education Council of the U.S. (SIECUS) recommend sex education that teaches: "Some common sexual behaviors shared by partners include kissing, touching, caressing, massaging, sharing erotic literature or art, bathing or showering together" (Guidelines for Comprehensive Sexuality Education).

This educational philosophy ignores the clear, significant risks of both pregnancy and sexually transmitted diseases. This sexual activity, usually called *foreplay,* is not safe. Sexual secretions can contain STD germs and foreplay often leads to intercourse. Foreplay is for the purpose of increasing the sexual interest between two people so they will progress into penetrative sexual intercourse. These activities will almost always arouse both partners to the extent that intercourse is inevitable. It is not right to teach young people to participate in this activity outside of marriage. If the implication is that STDs and pregnancy can be avoided with this activity, that is a false assumption. Disease organisms can survive in moist conditions outside the body long enough for infection to occur. The significance of broken skin must be understood. Even a small crack or cut or a skin rash can be an entryway to the body for STD. Be especially aware of those conditions on the inner parts of the thighs or hands. Understand that persons who have oral sex can get all the sexually transmitted diseases by that activity just as quickly as they can with vaginal intercourse.

If a young person has not learned how to say no to such activity, he or she will find it easy to progress from outercourse or mutual masturbation to intercourse or oral sex. Something so immediately pleasurable as uncommitted sex can feel like a huge magnet sucking one away from all the important things of life. Such sexual activity is not healthy and appropriate for unmarried persons. Those who would say so are betraying our youth. These intimate sexual acts belong only in marriage.

Life is more than just having sex. Yes, sex is an important part of life but it must be kept in balance with the rest of life or it can overwhelm other important areas: friendship, sports, family time, helping the less fortunate, and many other activities.

13

condoms

Do you really want to trust your future to a thin sheet of latex rubber?

Condoms do not give adequate protection for a woman's fertility.

Condoms give little, if any, protection against HPV, the most common STD in America.

The opportunities we have in the future depend on what we do today. Our conduct today will do something to us—either good or bad. We cannot escape that truth.

What does that truth have to do with the discussion of condoms? Simply this: Persons who become infected with STDs may become sterile, especially if they are female. A death sentence awaits those—male or female—who become HIV infected. There often is no second chance if STD damage occurs. Some of life's opportunities may be gone forever.

If you, as an unmarried person have intercourse with a partner who has had sexual intercourse one or more times with another person, you could become infected with an STD. You cannot escape that future possibility. It is the truth.

But wait—some experts will say that you can use a condom to decrease your chance of becoming infected. Years ago this was called *safe sex*. Now that they have seen the results of condom failure, they use the term *safer sex*.

My question, therefore, is: Do you really want to trust your future to a thin sheet of latex rubber? Your answer could affect your entire life. Do you want to be separated from disease or death by only a thin sheet of latex? What will you do if the latex has a hole or two, breaks during intercourse, or slips off during intercourse or withdrawal?

If you have sex as an unmarried person and your sex partner has an STD, you must use condoms correctly every single time you have intercourse to have any chance of protection. Even then, realize that condoms give almost no protection against HPV infection and give very inadequate protection for a woman's fertility. Even worse, remember that if the condom breaks or slips off, you have lost all protection and have significant risk of pregnancy or of becoming infected. Condoms, even if used correctly and consistently, cannot give you a 100 percent guarantee that you will not move from the safe side to the risk side. You can have a 100 percent guarantee only if you avoid sex until marriage and marry an uninfected partner.

That's it. That's the choice.

failure to prevent transmission of STDs

HPV

Listen to what some authorities say:

"Indeed, several studies have shown that condoms do not protect against this virus [HPV]."–Dr. Kenneth Noller, chairman of obstetrics and gynecology, University of Massachusetts School of Medicine.

"Condoms are useless in preventing HPV transmission because the virus is spread by cells that are shed onto the scrotum, which then come in contact with vulvar skin."–Michael Campion, director of gynecologic endoscopy, Graduate Hospital, Philadelphia.

Condoms, at best, offer only slight protection from human papillomavirus if one of the partners is infected (see chapter

5). Almost half of some groups of people who have had sexual intercourse outside of marriage are infected with HPV. Knowing that there is a 30 to 45 percent possibility of a sex partner having an HPV infection if he or she has had sex before, do you want to take a chance on a condom giving you protection against that disease? Are you willing to live with the consequences if it fails to protect you?

diseases that affect a woman's fertility

Some evidence suggests that condoms do not seem to provide good protection for a young woman's fertility (for example, an article by Samuels in the December 1989 *Medical Aspects of Human Sexuality*). No one knows exactly why. It may be because chlamydia mixes in all the sexual secretions and is therefore easily transmitted from one sex partner to another. It may be because chlamydia is so common that if a woman changes sex partners even two or three times over a period of years, she will have a high risk of becoming infected. About 50 to 80 percent of people currently infected with an STD are unaware of their infection because they have no symptoms of infection. Chlamydia and gonorrhea (see chapters 3 and 4) are sneaky diseases that can damage a woman's childbearing organs even when no symptoms are apparent. Since studies have so clearly confirmed that condoms did not give adequate protection for a woman's fertility, do you want to trust a thin sheet of latex to protect your own precious fertility—your ability to ever have a child?

HIV

Even when condoms are used correctly every time you have intercourse, you can still become infected with HIV. These are just two of the studies that indicate condoms are not effective in preventing HIV.

A 1995 study done by Johns Hopkins School of Medicine in Brazil showed that of 162 women who had sex with HIV positive men, 31 developed HIV in spite of the fact that they always used condoms.

Another study done by Dr. Susan Weller from the University of Texas School of Medicine showed that condoms had an average of 31 percent failure rate in preventing the transmission of HIV from an infected partner to an uninfected partner.

pregnancy prevention

Now that you understand that condoms cannot guarantee protection against STDs, why would you choose to use them? There is another risk. If you neglect to use a condom one time and it is at the "right time of the month," pregnancy can occur. When sperm are ejaculated into a woman's vagina, they can live in the cervical mucus for two or three days.

Almost all studies show that during the first year of using condoms to prevent pregnancy, ten to twenty women out of every one hundred become pregnant. Similar pregnancy rates exist for the second and third year of condom use.

what is the problem with condoms?

love interferes with condom use

When you are attracted to someone and you decide you would like to have intercourse, you probably do not see that person as someone who has sexually transmitted germs lurking inside a beautiful body. Remember, if that person has had sex with anyone in the past, he or she may be loaded with germs, germs that can infect you and change the future course of your life.

Perhaps you start out using condoms for protection but after a few weeks decide that such a wonderful person could not possibly be infected with an STD. Then you will probably stop using condoms and lose what little temporary protection they may have been providing. Condoms are not pleasant to use, they are inconvenient, and you decide that you really do not need all that protection. Then because that person was unaware of having an STD or was dishonest, you become infected. Does this happen often? Yes, it does. Do you really think you can trust your health to someone who doesn't commit to you for a lifetime?

Don't fool yourself: If you know you will not or do not use condoms every time you have sex, you cannot trust condoms.

Not one of us is perfect, and even our best resolutions often fail. A recent study of a group of HIV infected patients in Europe revealed that even though their sex partners were aware of the HIV infection, knew they were part of an intensive study, and knew the risks should they become infected, 123 out of 245 sex partners could not make themselves use condoms consistently and correctly over a period of two years. In that short period of time 12.7 percent became HIV infected. These were adult patients in stable relationships. Do you think you could do better?

no symptoms of STDs are apparent

You might feel comfortable not using condoms because your sex partner has no symptoms or signs of an STD. That lack of symptoms is merely setting a trap for you. From 50 to 80 percent of people infected with STDs do not know it because they have no signs or symptoms.

dishonest sexual partners

You may plan to use condoms if you have sex with someone who has had several other sex partners or with someone who is infected with a sexually transmitted disease. You might "interview" a potential sex partner who denies ever having sex with anyone else, who claims not to have had sex for a long, long time, or who denies having any disease. You might then have intercourse with that person. After a time, because things seem safe, you might become complacent and fail to use condoms reliably. Then because that other person was dishonest, you could become infected with an STD.

Almost all surveys of unmarried sexually active people reveal that many will lie about how many sex partners they have had. They will also lie about currently having another sex partner if they really want to have sex with you. The worst thing they can think of is being denied sex by you, and they know you might turn them down if you know their true story.

condom breakage and slippage

These are conservative statistics. Many other studies show even less condom reliability. One study of 106 women reported that 36 percent had experienced one condom breakage. The women reported further that 5 percent of their unplanned pregnancies could be traced to condom breakage. (These figures are taken from an article in *Contraception*, 1991.)

> 1.7 percent of condoms break during intercourse.
> 6.2 percent of condoms slip off during intercourse.
> 6.7 percent of condoms slip off during withdrawal.

When the condom breaks, all safety will fall, to paraphrase a nursery rhyme. Is this enough protection for you?

condom pores and holes

Some experts would say that few HIV organisms would leak through these defects. Even if only a few leak through, however, HIV infection could occur. One study demonstrated leakage of HIV-sized particles through pores in latex condoms in as many as twenty-nine of eighty-nine condoms. These pores are a normal result of the manufacturing process and are always present in latex. Would a thin sheet of latex be enough protection from HIV for you?

> Manufacturers may sell condoms that
> have 3 or 4 holes per 1,000 condoms.
>
> Condoms have 50–micron pores;
> HIV organism is .1 micron.
>
> Leakage of HIV–sized particles was found
> in as many as 29 out of 89 condoms.

condoms do not cover the entire body

Condoms cannot cover a painless syphilis sore at the top of a penis or on lips or tongues. A man may know he has a sore but if it doesn't hurt, he may think it could not be an STD. In the dark of night, he can put his condom on, his partner would know he had it on and be glad he was so responsible. However, she could get syphilis from contact with that painless sore if it is on his penis above the condom. Herpes and other STDs that cause ulcers can be passed to an unsuspecting sex partner any time an ulcer touches even a tiny break in the skin. Oral sex can transmit any STD. Therefore, condoms do not make sex safe. They cannot cover the whole body.

condoms do not cover the heart

Neither can condoms cover the emotional pain from broken relationships, from flashbacks of previous sexual activity, from a feeling of being used, or from disease that makes its victims feel dirty. Condoms do not protect against any of this emotional injury.

Don't lie to yourself. If you know you do not have the discipline to use condoms every single time you have sex, accept the fact that you will probably become either infected or pregnant. Also, accept the fact that some diseases may infect you even if you use your condoms correctly.

Consider the reasons condoms may and will fail you. Do not trust your entire future to a simple little piece of latex rubber. Your life is worth more than that—far more than that. Save sex for marriage; that is the only safe sex.

14

mutual monogamy
cohabitation before marriage

SHORT, MUTUAL MONOGAMOUS RELATIONSHIPS DO NOT
GIVE PROTECTION FROM STDs.

STATISTICS SHOW THAT COHABITATION BEFORE MARRIAGE
IS A DISASTER FOR TWO PEOPLE.

SOME PEOPLE BELIEVE THAT A MUTUALLY MONOGAMOUS
relationship can make sex safe. Such a relationship can allow
intimacy without entanglement. Mutual monogamy, a loose
relationship of cohabiting with a person of the opposite sex,
or trial marriage are names given to this lifestyle.

Ask yourself these questions if you are considering entering a mutually monogamous relationship:

1. What does monogamy mean—staying with one person
   for six months, a year, two years, five years?
2. When will I know that this monogamous relationship
   has lasted long enough and it is time to break it off?
3. How will I know it is time to start another monogamous relationship?
4. How many times can I change partners and still be safe
   so that when I enter marriage I will not have been damaged by STDs?

People who make the decision to begin having sex together
in a monogamous relationship generally do not plan to break

up in only a few months. Most of the time, however, they do. The relationship usually falls apart because infatuation and sex are not enough to keep two people together. The glue of commitment to the other person as a person is required for a relationship to survive. When a couple breaks up, each will often enter into a sexual relationship with the next person he or she feels attracted to. Mutually monogamous relationships of this type typically last from a few months to a couple of years.

If this has been your experience, you may look back and realize that, for example, you had sex with three or four people during your four years in college. If you have had this lifestyle, you need to be tested for STDs now, because this type of monogamy does not protect against them. In fact, monogamy of this type has caused the spread of STDs in the U.S. because the sharing of sexual secretions with several different people causes it. It doesn't make any difference whether the sexual contact with different people is made all in one night or over a period of five or more years. As far as the germs are concerned, they can be spread later as well as sooner.

cohabitation

You may not feel good about entering into casual sexual relationships of mutual monogamy. You may decide to move in with someone special without the commitment of marriage. This is commonly called *cohabitation.* Now that so many people in our society have tried cohabitation before marriage, researchers have been able to document its impact on couples. You may be surprised at some of the findings.

First, cohabitating couples have more problems in their relationships than married couples do.

Next, many cohabitating couples break up before they marry. One researcher found this happened to 40 percent of the couples he studied. Although cohabitating couples are not married, the ending of the relationship is often as emotionally devastating as a divorce.

Even if cohabitating couples marry, they have more problems than couples who were married before entering into a sexual relationship. Studies show cohabitating couples have greater marital conflict and poorer communication than couples who married before cohabitating. Couples who engaged in sex before marriage were more likely to commit adultery in their marriage than those who waited until marriage to engage in sex.

Finally, couples who cohabit before marriage have a 50 percent higher divorce rate than those who did not cohabit before their wedding.

Consider it an insult for someone to want to have sex with you without marrying you. If someone cares enough about you as a person to have sex, that person should care enough about you to want to spend the rest of his or her life with you. Anything short of that is an affront to you as an intact, whole, worthy individual. It is saying to you that the other person would like to receive sexual pleasure from you with no commitment, with no responsibility, and with hesitation about being truly committed to you as a person. Even worse, that person wants you to enter into a relationship that is far more likely to be unhappy and destructive to both of you than a marriage relationship.

Marriage has received a bad rap in the past few years. Modern research has shown it to be a much more fulfilling relationship than it receives credit for. A statement in the book *Sex in America* is interesting:

> The relationship between being married and having orgasms during sex with a partner was very strong. Married women had much higher rates of usually or always having orgasm. . . . Those having the most partnered-sex and enjoying it the most are the married people. . . . In real life, the unheralded, seldom discussed world of married sex is actually one that satisfies people the most.
>
> Michael, Gagnon, Laumann, and Kolta (Boston: Little, Brown and Company, 1994), 127.

15

uncommitted sex and emotional health

"IT IS ACCEPTABLE FOR A MAN TO FORCE SEX ON A WOMAN IF THEY HAVE BEEN DATING FOR SIX MONTHS OR MORE." IN A RHODE ISLAND SURVEY OF MIDDLE SCHOOL STUDENTS 65% OF BOYS AND 49% OF GIRLS AGREED TO THAT STATEMENT.

HIGH SCHOOL STUDENTS WITH SEVERAL SEX PARTNERS WERE MORE LIKELY TO HAVE GREATER FREQUENCY AND SEVERITY OF RECENT AND LIFETIME DRUG USE THAN STUDENTS WHO DO NOT ENGAGE IN SEXUAL ACTIVITY. (FROM A STUDY BY HARVARD MEDICAL SCHOOL, 1995.)

APPROXIMATELY 25% OF AMERICAN WOMEN, AGE 20 AND UNDER, ARE SEXUALLY ABUSED.

A LARGE NUMBER OF MEN HAVE BEEN SEXUALLY PRESSURED BY WOMEN.

PEOPLE WHO HAVE BEEN SEXUALLY ABUSED BEFORE AGE 16 BY SOMEONE MORE THAN 5 YEARS OLDER HAVE A SIGNIFICANTLY INCREASED INCIDENCE OF SUICIDE ATTEMPTS AND EATING DISORDERS.

IF YOUNG PEOPLE BECOME INVOLVED IN SEXUAL ACTIVITY, THEY GENERALLY PERFORM MORE POORLY IN SCHOOL AND HAVE LOWER EDUCATIONAL ASPIRATIONS.

ALTHOUGH IT IS HARD TO KNOW WHICH IS THE CAUSE AND which is the effect of these problems, sexual activity by young people is clearly associated with disturbing emotional problems. The examples given above show how emotionally hurt young people can be by inappropriate sexual activity. Neither the abused nor their abusers feel good about themselves. The Rhode Island young people have had their perception of sexuality so damaged that they think it is normal, even acceptable, to be forced to have sexual intercourse.

A result of this terribly misunderstood sexuality is apparent in this paragraph from a letter I received from one of my patients who had been sexually active when she was young.

> What people fail to understand is that when a person has sex with someone they give a part of themselves away to that other person. To do this over and over again with multiple partners chips away at a healthy self-esteem and self-respect. That person is left feeling empty, lonely, and worthless. This is what happened to me, and I would resort to sex again to combat the overwhelming emptiness and loneliness I felt. It was a vicious cycle.

Several years ago a teenager was a patient of mine. She had already been sexually active. Later, when she was thirty-five she moved back to town. I asked her about her past history of sexual activity. She said she had hated every minute of it. She would even think about it when taking a shower. She remembered her first act of intercourse and felt how terrible that experience was. Her strong recommendation to teenagers is that they not get involved in sex until they get married. Premarital sexual activity is "something that literally stays with a person for an entire lifetime."

Dick Pernell, a counselor, says that he hears "over and over about the guilt and emptiness and regret people experience after uncommitted sex." What they say usually goes something like this: "At first it was very, very exciting. Then I started to feel bad about myself. Then I started to feel bad about the person I was with. We started to argue and fight a lot. Then we broke up and now we are enemies."

In a radio interview, clinical psychologist Dr. Kevin Leman describes the "sexual flashbacks" that trouble a number of the married women he has counseled. Another expert confirms the reality of these flashbacks:

> When they make love with their husbands, they suffer—sometimes ten or fifteen years into the marriage—involuntary mental images of premarital sex with other partners. Men are also vulnerable to these disruptive flashbacks. Says one young husband: "I am married to one of the most wonderful women I have ever met. I would do anything for her. And I would do anything, anything, to forget the sexual experiences I had before I met my wife. When we start having intercourse, the pictures of the past and the other women go through my mind, and it is killing any intimacy. I am to the point I do not want to have sex because I can't stand those memories. The truth is I have been married to this wonderful woman for eight years and I have never been 'alone' in the bedroom with her."
>
> From *Educating for Character,* Thomas Lickona
> (New York: Bantam, 1991), 336–8

These personal catastrophes could happen to you. The problems changed the lives of the people involved—for the worse. You can avoid the pain they experienced by postponing sexual intercourse until marriage. If you have been sexually abused, see a counselor. If you, as a single person, have an overwhelming desire to engage in sexual activity, see a counselor to determine why you might have this destructive compulsion.

16

say no—why and how

THE ENCHANTMENT, LOVE, AND ROMANCE OF THE TEENAGE YEARS CAN BE DESTROYED BY GIVING IN TO LEADEN, OBLIGATORY, MECHANICAL SEX.

FIFTEEN-YEAR-OLDS WITH TEN OR MORE "PARTNERS" DO NOT MERELY FAIL TO FIND LOVE; THEY ALSO FAIL TO FIND PLEASURE, FOR THEY ARE ALMOST NEVER ORGASMIC.

PREMARITAL SEXUAL ACTIVITY IS OFTEN MERELY ANOTHER FORM OF SEXUAL ABUSE.

WHY SHOULD YOU SAY NO TO SEXUAL ACTIVITY UNTIL YOU ARE married? One reason is that sexual activity will often destroy the romance, enchantment, and mystery of the married relationship between a man and a woman. There is no way to make certain an out-of-wedlock pregnancy or infection with an STD will not occur if you are having sexual intercourse with someone who has had sex with someone else.

The greatest risk is having more than one sex partner. When you marry, you commit to having only one sex partner for life. If any diseases affect either of you, you can deal with them together.

why singles want to have intercourse

not only for pleasure

Sharon Thomson, author of *Going All the Way—Teenage Girls' Tales of Sex, Romance, and Pregnancy,* found that the majority of all girls who engage in sexual intercourse do not do it because they feel desire for a guy or because they thought it would give them great pleasure. Generally they did it to achieve some other goal. Often it was trading sex for "true love." Others did it as an act of rebellion against parents or other authorities in their lives. (From an interview quoted in "Family Life Matters," newsletter, Rutgers University, Winter 1996.)

the past sexual abuse factor

Experts say that about 22 percent of women in America have been forced to do something sexually against their will or that they did not like. Women who have been sexually abused will often be sexually promiscuous later. This problem does not affect only women. One 1994 report pointed out that one out of three predominately heterosexual male college students had experienced an incident of being forced or pressured to have sex after age sixteen. For at least 22 percent of the men, the encounter resulted in genital or oral intercourse. About 20 percent of the men had such a strong negative reaction that they worried if they were abnormal for having refused easy sex. (C. and D. Struckman-Johnson, *Archives of Sexual Behavior,* 23:93, February 1994).

peer pressure

Peer pressure is commonly a reason for teenagers to begin sexual activity. Young people who believe their friends at school are engaging in sexual activity think they would be shamed or shunned if they were not also having sex.

One young couple was kidded so incessantly about being virgins that they decided to have sex one time. Not because they wanted to, but they thought if they were no longer virgins, the kidding would stop. With this first and only act of intercourse, the young woman became pregnant.

Consider this type of peer pressure as illegal, immoral, and wrong. Do not put up with it. Enlist the help of school administrators or parents to help get the pressure stopped.

loneliness and lack of intimacy

Many young men and women engage in sexual intercourse because they are lonely. Maybe parents are not home or are too busy to pay attention to their children. If you are thinking about having sexual intercourse because you feel lonely, tell a parent or a trusted friend about your feelings. He or she can help you find love in another, more healthy way. Having sexual intercourse because you are lonely will not solve your loneliness problem. It will cause you even worse problems of loneliness, depression, and feelings of shame, especially if you become infected with an STD or become pregnant.

drugs and alcohol

Drugs and/or alcohol tend to lower inhibitions against sexual intercourse. One study reported that 60 percent of college women who acquired an STD were drunk at the time of the infection. It also reported that 90 percent of rapes which occur on college campuses happen when one or both of the parties have used alcohol.

sex with older people

Men older than high school age account for 77 percent of all births among girls ages sixteen to eighteen and for 51 percent of births among girls age fifteen and younger.

Men over age twenty-five father twice as many teenage births as do boys under age eighteen.

Men over age twenty father five times more births among junior high girls than do junior high boys, and two and one-half times more births among senior high school age girls than do senior high school age boys.

Junior high boys account for 7 percent of births among junior high girls. Senior high boys father 24 percent of births among all school age girls.

Adult women over age twenty account for 14 percent of births fathered by school age boys.

The younger the mother, the greater the age gap. When the mother is twelve years old or younger, the father averages twenty-two years of age; when the mother is junior high age, the father is nearly five years older. When the mother is high school age, the father is nearly four years older.

While these figures are from a study done in California, they have profound implications for all of us. STD and AIDS rates are 2.5 times higher in females than they are in males under age twenty. This "surplus" points strongly to transmission from older men.

great relationships—without sex

Men and women of any age can (and do!) have healthy, happy relationships that do not include sexual activity until marriage.

Magazines, newspapers, television, movies, and videos often subtly yet strongly suggest that sex is a central aspect of almost all conversations and interaction between men and women, and that ultimately any man and woman who have the slightest attraction to each other will, if they are normal, have sexual intercourse. All of this is false and dishonest. Men and women of any age are not abnormal if they do not have sexual intercourse; they can (and do!) have healthy, happy relationships that do not include sexual activity until marriage.

These recommendations will help you have great interaction (without sex) with a person of the opposite sex.

1. Find a good friend with the same resolve about sex. One of my acquaintances recalled that during her teenage years she had a close girl friend with whom she shared the same values. They kept each other out of trouble. Whenever one would weaken, the other would be strong. Such a close friend can be invaluable. Even if a man drops you because you will not have sex with him, you will have a caring friend ready to help you pick up the pieces.

2. Write out your decision about sex. Put this reminder where you can see it every day, especially if you are undergoing a period of temptation. Keep reviewing it.

3. Practice assertiveness. Many people meekly surrender their independence when someone pressures them into doing something they know is wrong. If your moral decisions are being challenged, it's time to be assertive. Every person has the right to make decisions concerning his or her own body, especially when one's health is at stake. It is also important to realize that the mind and heart can control the body's urges.

4. Let your values be known to the man or woman with whom you share a mutual attraction. It is important for one with whom you are becoming increasingly romantically involved to know that you are not going to have intercourse until you marry. That knowledge can also be a weapon against date rape. No one can misinterpret your dress, smile, and gentle touch as signals that you want to have sex. Early in a relationship be assertive enough about your intention so that your date understands that no means no, not try again later.

5. Do not get involved with a man or woman you suspect will try to have sex with you. Sometimes it is very clear that a date is more interested in your physical self than in you as a total person. Remember your resolve and get rid of him or her.

6. Plan your dates and allow minimal time for uninterrupted privacy. Don't just "get together" and see what

happens. That is when you are most likely to end up having unwanted sex. Many people who become involved in sex did not mean to; they merely had no particular plans for the evening, and intercourse resulted.

7. Avoid using alcohol and drugs. Many men use these substances to get a woman into bed. Occasionally women do the same thing to have sex with a man. Alcohol and drugs deaden the mind and resolve. Stay away from them.

8. Have your dates meet your parents. It is healthy for your dates to know that your parents value you and want you to be treated as a person of worth.

9. Group date. Dating with others dramatically decreases time alone with one person of the opposite sex which in turn decreases temptation.

10. Limit the amount of physical contact. If you have said no but allow a man to have some freedom with your breasts or access into your clothes, he is going to think you really do want to have intercourse. You, the woman, must set the limits. You have that right. Once you allow a man certain privileges with your body, even well-intentioned and otherwise moral men will often forceably try to proceed all the way to intercourse and you may not be able to stop them because men are almost always stronger than women. Set a restrictive standard for physical contact early in your relationship.

The activities which should be avoided until marriage are:

Unfastening or unbuttoning clothing.
Removing articles of clothing.
Touching underneath clothing.
Kissing passionately for extended periods of time.
Lying down and passionately caressing each other.
Producing genital arousal on purpose.

One guideline I have recommended to single people is that they never allow another person to touch them anywhere their underwear touches them—either over their clothing or under their clothing.

11. Make a self-discipline pact. If you are a young person, ask your parents to set a time for you to come in. You may suggest that your parents wait up for you until you come in from a date. Older single persons can do the same thing and ask a roommate to wait up for them. Set limits that will allow you to have guidelines for the length of time you are with another person on a date and an end for that period of time. This time limit can stop passion that might be developing.

There is fun, joy, pleasure, romance, and enchantment in life. You can enjoy them by keeping your relationships with people of the opposite sex free of sexual involvement until marriage.

17

secondary virginity

THE GREATEST RISK FOR BECOMING INFECTED WITH AN STD IS HAVING SEVERAL SEX PARTNERS IN YOUR LIFETIME.

THE SECOND GREATEST RISK FOR BECOMING INFECTED WITH AN STD IS BEGINNING INTERCOURSE AT A YOUNG AGE.

SECONDARY VIRGINITY, OR STOPPING ALL SEXUAL INTERCOURSE UNTIL MARRIAGE, CAN INCREASE THE CHANCE OF BEING FREE FROM THE DISASTERS OF A SEXUALLY TRANSMITTED DISEASE AND OUT-OF-WEDLOCK PREGNANCY BECAUSE IT LIMITS THE NUMBER OF LIFETIME SEX PARTNERS.

IF YOU ARE NOT MARRIED AND ARE HAVING SEXUAL INTERCOURSE, STOP NOW! I mean to sound pushy! I want to send a clear message! Why? Recent research clearly shows that premarital intercourse is a prescription for disaster. The fewer sex partners one has during a lifetime, the greater the chance of remaining free from STDs. Avoiding sex until marriage also eliminates the intense emotional costs of premarital sex.

How can abstinence, or secondary virginity, possibly help a future marriage? Let me answer that by asking two questions:

Does the one you are having sex with really love you for who you are, or just for the sexual pleasure you provide him or her?

Will that person agree to a decision to be abstinent from now until both of you decide if marriage is right for the two of you and the wedding takes place?

If both partners agree to the abstinence agreement, each has been honored in an extravagant way by the other. Choosing abstinence shows that the partners view each other not just as sex objects but as respected and loved human beings. To receive this degree of respect and integrity from another person can generate a love in you that you did not know you were capable of. This type of mutual love, trust, and honesty lays a foundation for marriage that will help build and maintain a strong and safe future marriage.

> The fewer sex partners one has during a lifetime, the greater the chance of remaining free from STDs.

If your sex partner will not agree to abstinence until marriage, I encourage you to find a friend to stand by you as you terminate the relationship. A friend can help hear your cries of loneliness and heal a broken heart. The loneliness is usually felt most by the woman in the relationship because she realizes that if the man will not agree to be abstinent until marriage, he was probably interested in her only for sexual pleasure. Although the separation hurts deeply, broken hearts do heal, especially with the help of friends.

As you heal, you will become increasingly aware that yours had been an emotionally unhealthy relationship. Now begin looking for a person who respects and loves you for who you are—not just for your vagina or your penis.

If you cannot end the present sexual relationship, at least make the decision that if this relationship does break up, you will not start having sex with the next person you get close to. Make that decision now as you remember that the more sex partners you have in your lifetime, the greater the chance you have for contracting an STD.

A patient of mine has some words for you:

We were taught in the high school health classes about contraceptives and sexually transmitted diseases. The impression

I was getting from adults was that it was totally O.K. and acceptable to engage in premarital sex as long as you did it safely.

I felt proud to be a liberated young woman—a step above the rest because I was free from restrictions and self-restraint. So I openly and frequently engaged in sex with many different partners, some of whom were unknown to me. I grew popular among the boys. I enjoyed being desired and I enjoyed sex.

What I didn't realize in the beginning was that I was being used. I became more aware of this when at times I would turn down the advances of a boy and suffer cruel rejection. What was worse though, was the rejection suffered after I slept with them. But I usually gave the boys what they wanted so they would like me. I covered up my own pain by convincing myself that I was using them for my own sexual pleasure. I did enjoy sex but there were terrible consequences which I did not attribute to premarital sex until looking back.

. . . when I first became sexually active at age fifteen, I insisted on using condoms, but I soon discovered that they were uncomfortable and inconvenient for myself and for my partner especially. Guys hate condoms. . . . Then I tried oral contraceptives which were given to me by Planned Parenthood, but I was too irresponsible to remember to take them consistently. These, also, did not offer any protection against sexually transmitted diseases, which I would later learn for myself from firsthand experience. But, like most teenagers, I never thought it could happen to me.

Aside from the physical consequences, there were devastating spiritual and psychological consequences as well, that were not as obvious. . . . I began to spiral down into hopelessness and despair leading to suicidal tendencies. What people fail to understand is that when a person has sex with someone, they give a part of themselves away to that other person. To do this over and over again with multiple partners chips away at a healthy self-esteem and self-respect. That person is left feeling empty, lonely, and worthless. This is what happened to me. Being ignorant of this, I would resort to sex again to combat the overwhelming emptiness and loneliness I felt. It was a vicious cycle. . . .

You had asked that I write you about my past sexual history, being that I was once quite promiscuous, but I've been celibate the last five years. . . . I look forward to my honeymoon night with my new husband (in February). . . . I was a slave to the promiscuous lifestyle.

Abstinence is freedom. I am now a truly liberated woman. Thank you, Dr. M., for all your efforts to teach our young people about abstinence. How I wish I could have been exposed to your values when I was a teenager. Perhaps I would have made some better choices if I had known there was an alternative.

This patient experienced the freedom of secondary virginity. You can experience it too! It is an extremely difficult decision to make and an even harder one to stick to. You can do both and experience the joy of freedom from being a slave to sexual entanglement. You can enjoy a truly liberated life now and in the future.

18

25, 35, 45— still single and celibate?

"IF YOU DON'T USE IT, YOU WILL LOSE IT"—WRONG

"EVERYONE ELSE IS HAVING SEXUAL INTERCOURSE"—WRONG

"SEXUAL INTERCOURSE OUTSIDE A LIFELONG COMMITMENT TO AND FROM A PARTNER IS ONLY A CHARADE OF INTIMACY"—RIGHT

SINGLE, CELIBATE PEOPLE IN THEIR MIDDLE TO LATE TWENTIES or older can feel left out in the cold when discussions of sex come up.

Single, sexually involved people may acknowledge that the STD risk does concern them but they are not about to stop having intercourse.

Single, celibate people may feel they are condemned to a life without intimacy. They have denied themselves something in which even many junior high and senior high school students indulge.

Abstaining from sexual intercourse or becoming celibate again after a broken relationship or divorce is a perplexing experience for an adult.

The ideas in this chapter may help you chart a course that will keep you out of sexually troubled waters during the next few years.

popular misconceptions

Today's teenagers reach physical maturity earlier and marry later. There has been a steady increase in the percentage of young people having sexual intercourse, and in the percentage, doing so at younger and younger ages. Almost all teenagers experiment with some type of sexual behavior.

> *Facing Facts: Sexual Health for America's Adolescents,*
> Debra W. Haffner, ed. (New York: [SIECUS]
> Sexuality Information and Education Council
> of the United States, 1995), 1.

The clear implication is that human physiology now mandates sexual activity. Since maturity is so early and marriage is so late, people will, therefore, inevitably engage in sexual activity. "It's in the genes." The best response to these notions is "Not true," or a word teenagers used frequently in the early nineties: "*NOT!*"

alarming facts

Human sexuality is much more special, much more comprehensive than a mere physiologic imperative. That philosophy describes animals, not adult men and women. Granted, there is a lot of time from physiologic maturity until marriage. Granted, you may be one of the people in the U.S. who will never be married. That is precisely why you should not begin sexual activity until—and if—you enter into a lifelong monogamous relationship with a faithful partner, a relationship called marriage.

For example, if you begin having sex with different people at age sixteen and get married at age nineteen, you would have time to have only a few sex partners—unless you are very promiscuous. However, if you begin having sex at age sixteen, have different partners periodically, and do not marry until you are age twenty-eight, you would have time to have many more sex partners (even if you were not what is considered promiscuous) than if you had married at age nineteen. Premarital sex is a dangerous lifestyle because all studies show that the possibilities of contracting an STD increase dramatically with the addition of each sex partner during one's lifetime.

current misunderstandings

There seems to be misunderstanding about this issue among singles and those who are single again after a divorce or death. After a talk I gave about women's hormones at a meeting, a forty-year-old woman asked if we could talk privately for a minute. She had chosen to be abstinent since she was divorced ten years previously. Her friends were telling her it was unhealthy for her to remain abstinent. They used the phrase: "If you don't use it, you'll lose it." I assured her that statement was untrue and encouraged her to continue to be abstinent until marriage.

Misinformation about STDs seems common among older single people. One reason may be that older single people tend to think that STDs are a teenage problem and "cannot happen to me." Another reason may be that when these thirty something people grew up in the '60s and '70s, the incidence of sexually transmitted disease was much lower than it is now. It is almost impossible for them to accept the fact that today anyone who has had several sex partners is probably infected with an STD.

Let's review a few statistics already given:

The number one reason for the death of Americans age 25–45 is AIDS.

Herpes infects at least 30 percent of sexually active single people by age 30.

Chlamydia is found in 10–30 percent of sexually active single people.

Clearly the STD epidemic has made major inroads into the single, sexually active community. Pregnancy is also a common, major problem for sexually active singles. The highest percentage of pregnant women having an abortion are those age forty and over—a commentary on how many women that age get pregnant and don't want to be.

There is a great deal of societial pressure on older single people to become sexually involved. The majority of their peers are married. Many older singles have been married and obviously participated in sexual activity in those marriages. It is difficult to become celibate again once sexual activity has been a part of one's life.

Single people frequently find society a somewhat hostile environment. Acquaintances may assume that a celibate person is lesbian or gay. The world seems to be organized for couples. Singles may feel misunderstood or feel the absence of intimacy and may try to fill that void with sexual activity.

Single people will often feel they are missing out on something. Obviously, they are missing out on having sexual intercourse if they are abstinent. Many of my single friends have told me that loneliness is one of the major problems of the single life. They are interested in sexual activity, not necessarily because of the physical pleasure they imagine they would get from it, but because of the intimacy it would bring to their lives. Intimacy is a valid need. All human beings need intimacy. Because sexual intercourse is such an intimate act, it would seem to provide the intimacy that single people desire.

true intimacy

SEXUAL INTERCOURSE OUTSIDE OF A LIFELONG COMMITMENT TO AND FROM A PARTNER IS ONLY A CHARADE OF INTIMACY. Many people who have sought intimacy by having sexual intercourse have found that not only does it not provide the intimacy they sought, but it also destroys communication, warmth, and commitment in the relationship. Women generally sense this destruction sooner than men because women usually enter into a sexual experience seeking love and closeness. Men often enter it for physical pleasure. But men also lose in this type of out-of-wedlock sexual relationship. Men learn intimacy and warmth from a lifetime commitment to a woman. They lose that in sexual relationships that are not permanent commitments.

The destruction of true intimacy by sexual contact outside of a lifelong commitment is an enigma, a conundrum, a paradox. I don't believe we will ever truly understand why sexual intercourse outside of marriage is so destructive, but it is. Not only is it destructive to the intimate emotional needs of the people involved, but even to the sex act itself. Listen to what the authors of *Sex in America* say:

> The least satisfied were those who were not married, not living with anyone, and who had at least two sex partners. Only 54 percent of them reported they were extremely or very physically pleased and only one-third said they were extremely or very emotionally satisfied. . . . Physical and emotional satisfaction started to decline when people had more than one sex partner. . . . The most suggestive number, however . . . is the fact that never married and non-cohabiting women have much higher rates of never having orgasms—11 percent—compared to the rates for all other women—2 percent.

The authors of *Sex in America* concluded: "In real life, the unheralded, seldom discussed world of married sex is actually the one that satisfies people the most." The principle that those who seek pleasure are the ones least likely to find it does apply to sexual activity outside of the marriage relationship.

Contrary to popular opinion, many single people are not sexually active. The authors of *Sex in America* reported on interviews with 3,432 scientifically selected individuals. Of those who were never married and not living with a person of the opposite sex, 12 percent had never had sexual intercourse.

The authors further say,

> The increase in the number of men who are virgins at age twenty began before the AIDS scare, so we cannot attribute all of that increase to concerns about AIDS. We are not certain why more twenty-year-olds are virgins now than forty years ago, and can only speculate that perhaps it has become more socially acceptable for a young man to refrain from having intercourse. We found, for example, that the proportion of men whose first sexual intercourse was with a prostitute declined from 7 percent of men who came of age in the 1950s to 1.5 percent of men who came of age in the 1980s to early 1990s. . . . The proportion of women who were virgins had traditionally been somewhat higher than the proportion of men who had had no sexual intercourse by age twenty, but that gender difference has disappeared.

celibacy—go for it

Just because you have friends who are not having sex and are still virgins does not mean it is easy for you to maintain your virginity or secondary virginity, but it certainly is comforting to know that there are others like you.

Realize that sex is a wonderful thing, but it has its balance in our lives only in a relationship with one other person for the long haul. This is called marriage. Although sex is a siren that calls loudly to you, it is a call that can be resisted. As you resist the call, you will be strengthened. You will have a life physically more healthy because you won't be infected with STDs. You won't have the pain of an out-of-wedlock pregnancy. You will have a life more emotionally whole because you won't be damaged by scars and memories of the past. If you are to be married, you will be able to look forward to a life more free from problems and pain, more able to do those things you want to do. I'm not saying it won't be a rocky road, but you can live a celibate life as a single person. What better gift to give yourself?

19

sexual activity
developing a personal code

NOW THAT YOU HAVE LOOKED AT SEXUALITY FROM MANY angles and know that it is both great and powerful, it is time to determine your personal code for sexual behavior. You face almost irresistible pressure to follow the powerful drive to have sexual intercourse. Will you allow it to eclipse the fragile and human part of sex?

Your life is packed with potential—potential for pleasure, for success—and for happiness. Hope alone will not make these things happen, but careful attention to your life can.

To keep your life healthy may require some hard choices now, may mean loss of some freedom now. But carefully guiding your life now by making good choices will help protect that potential for health, success, happiness, and for doing good that is inside you. The choice is yours. Choose wisely.

the funnel principle

The "funnel principle" may help you develop a personal code for sexual behavior. A funnel is narrow at one end and much wider at the other. Life is like a funnel and the funnel can work in one of two ways. You have a choice about how you use it.

The first way is to do anything you want—whatever looks right or good to you today, limited only by your desires.

This is experiencing life in the wide open end of the funnel. There are no restraints. There is freedom to do whatever you decide to do.

There is a problem with this behavior. Later you may find yourself living life in the narrow end of the funnel. Your opportunities have been narrowed down, leaving you with fewer choices and with more problems than you had expected.

For example, your choice as a single woman might be to have intercourse with a boyfriend because you are in love or perhaps just because you want to. This is life in the free, no limits, wide open end of the funnel. One result of this choice might be an infection with chlamydia that results in your sterility. Later, when you are married, you could discover that you are unable to become pregnant and you could spend enormous amounts of time, money, and emotions exploring possible options that might allow you to become pregnant. This is life in the narrow, limited end of the funnel—fewer opportunities and more trouble—a direct result of your previous choices.

What happens if you turn the funnel over and enter the narrow end first? You limit your choices now because those limits will make your life better in the future. You may, for example, practice the self-discipline of not having sex until marriage. This is entering the narrow end of the funnel first. The benefit will probably be that when you decide to get pregnant it will happen easily within only a few months of practicing normal intercourse. This is freedom.

Life offers you many future possibilities for happiness and fulfillment. Life can be better now and so much better in the future if you don't destroy your future opportunities by bad choices. Remember, there are some bridges that burn behind you, that keep you from going back and changing things. Some actions in life will give you no second chance. How can you plan for a truly meaningful, healthy sexuality that you can enjoy the rest of your life?

elements of healthy sexuality

Consider these four areas as you develop your personal code: self-esteem, faith, parental relationships, and future marriage partnership. Spend some time thinking about your future.

self – esteem

Your single friends may have begun having sex out of curiosity or because a long, close relationship finally resulted in intercourse. Many people, however, become sexually involved because they don't feel good about themselves. They have low self-esteem and have convinced themselves that love from another person will prove their self-worth. If sex is required to get that love, then sex is worth it. Avoid this trap. Having sex to gain self-esteem is not the answer. Often, instead of producing a happy feeling of good self-esteem, having sex results in poorer self-esteem, especially if it results in an STD infection or pregnancy.

All of us have some of the feelings listed below some of the time. If, however, you have some of these feelings most of the time, you are probably suffering from poor self-esteem.

1. I don't feel truly loved by at least one parent.
2. I don't feel appreciated or accepted by a parent.
3. I don't feel that at least one parent has time for me.
4. I don't have even one adult I respect with whom I can talk about important thoughts or feelings.
5. I feel inferior or worthless.
6. I feel that no one likes me; I feel all alone.
7. I feel that I rarely do anything right, or that I rarely do anything well.
8. I feel that I rarely do anything worthwhile, productive, or useful.
9. I feel that people usually disapprove of me, of my ideas, and of my morals.

10. I feel that I "must" do things I don't feel right about or that I don't really want to do because of pressure from others.
11. I feel that I must think of my own good all the time and not of the good of others.

If you are suffering from poor self-esteem, the first step is to ask a trusted family member, friend, or professional to help you deal with your feelings. He or she can help you begin to see yourself as the special person you are. Ultimately you will realize that since you have great worth, you are capable of making decisions for yourself that will help you to be healthy, happy, and successful in the future. You will have good character, good values, and good self-esteem. If you have been abused (physically, emotionally, sexually) in the past or are now in an abusive relationship, you too should seek out a friend, family member, or professional to help you deal with your feelings. Don't "stuff" your feelings or postpone getting help. You can overcome your negative feelings and fears.

faith

If faith in God is important to you, you have a better chance of having a fulfilling sexual life than people who do not hold a faith. Reliable research consistently shows that persons who believe in God have a much more satisfying sexual life than non-religious people.

Researchers were surprised when a *Redbook* magazine survey taken in the early 1970s (approximately 100,000 women involved) found that highly religious women described their sex lives as "good" or "very good" a significantly higher proportion of times than did non-religious women.

Tavrisc and Sadds evaluated these findings in *The Redbook Report on Female Sexuality* (N.Y.: Delacorte Press, 1977). They reported: "Higher proportions of the religious group reported to be orgasmic more often and more satisfied with the frequency of their sexual activity than their non-religious counterparts."

Other more recent studies have shown the same result. Michael, Gagnon, Laumann, and Kolta, researchers at the University of Chicago, reported in *Sex in America: A Definitive Survey* (1993):

> Women with no religious affiliation were somewhat less likely to report that they always had an orgasm, while the conservative Protestant women had the highest rates. . . . The association for women between religious affiliation and orgasm may seem surprising because conservative religious women are so often portrayed as sexually repressed. Perhaps conservative Protestant women firmly believe in the holiness of marriage and of sexuality as an expression of their love for their husbands. In this sense, the findings are consistent with the other findings on sexual satisfaction.

Studies now make it clear that religious people usually are not ashamed of sex. They enjoy it greatly, as a matter of fact, more so than any other group in the U.S. So the myth that religious men and women as a group are sexually neurotic and repressed is just that—a myth. Don't listen to the message currently taught by some organizations that young people should accept values that differ from the teachings of their faith. Keep your faith vibrant and strong. That will give you the best chance for a good sex life.

parents

Your parents (or parent) care more about you than anyone else in the entire world. They love you. When they give you direction, they are doing it for your benefit and protection, not to limit or hurt you. Friends come and go. So do teachers. Parents are family. They will usually be there to give you advice, guidance, and love after everyone else is gone. They are older, have had more of life's experiences, and are in the best position to see a little farther down the road of life than you can see.

They know that you are developing the ability to make good choices. They know that if you do not develop the maturity to make good choices in the future, you can be severely hurt by life. If you don't have the self-discipline to study when you are in high school or college, you may not be able to graduate and get a good job. If you don't have the self-discipline to keep yourself from having sex until marriage, you might become infected with a sexually transmitted disease that could permanently scar your life.

Your parents' job is to show you what good choices are. Their do's and don'ts can help you learn values that you can use in the future when you are making all your own decisions. It is hard for them to set limits and enforce them. It is sometimes hard for you to accept them. The personal moral strength you develop through their guidance can help in the long run and allow you more personal freedom.

Keep in mind that ultimately your parents' discipline, guidance, and limits are going to help you be the person your parents know you can be and the person you want to be.

marriage

Why is it best to wait until marriage to have sex? Societies have traditionally protected the marriage and family relationship with ferocious intensity. Societies know that one of the most important tasks they must accomplish if they want to survive is to do everything they can to encourage a man and a woman to stay together for life. The reason is that a stable family life is necessary for children to grow into adulthood and continue to pass on the pattern for a stable lifestyle.

Some societies in the past, and even today, feel strongly about keeping their families intact. Very strongly, in fact. Adultery and sex before marriage are, and were, often punished by stiff penalties and, in some cultures, by death.

In America marriage is honored with legal recognition by laws. We have also surrounded marriage with many symbols that show we regard it as a highly important relationship: the rings, the wedding dress, the marriage ceremony, gifts, and anniversary celebrations. All of these things say, "This is special and must be protected, not just for the good of the couple, but also for the good of society and culture."

What is so good about marriage? What does it accomplish that cannot be accomplished without such bothersome entanglement? Why should marriage be the goal you strive for if you want to be sexually involved someday? Why should you avoid sexual activity until that time? Marriage is the best place for sex because:

1. There is a decreased risk of sexually transmitted diseases when both marriage partners are committed to each other.
2. The possibility of out-of-wedlock pregnancy is eliminated when sex is postponed until marriage.
3. There is a lower rate of abuse of pregnant women. For every married pregnant woman who is abused by her husband, almost four unmarried pregnant women are abused by their partners. A study by the New Jersey State Police Uniform Crime Reporting Unit, reported in *1991 Domestic Violence Report,* indicates that being unmarried is the strongest predictor of abuse—stronger than race, educational attainment, housing conditions, or access to prenatal care.
4. Single mothers often face financial difficulties. Statistics indicate that single-parent families are six times more likely to be poor than married-couple families.
5. The recent highly acclaimed study by the University of Chicago reported: "Married women had much higher rates (75 percent) of usually or always having orgasms. . . . The young people who flit from partner to partner and seem to be having a sex life that is sattisfying beyond most people's dreams, are, it seems,

mostly a media creation. In real fact, the unheralded, seldom discussed, world of married sex is actually the one that satisfies people the most."

It is not necessary for an individual to be married or to be sexually active to be a complete and fulfilled person. Many of the world's most esteemed and respected individuals were not, or are not, married. Mother Teresa, and, until he married late in life, C. S. Lewis, are two contemporary examples of fulfilled single people. They affirm the importance to society of sexually abstinent, highly productive, praiseworthy individuals.

If you plan to become sexually involved, plan for your involvement to take place in marriage. If you have this goal and follow your dream, you will be more likely to be happy and healthy. You will have a greater chance to have babies. You will have fewer bad memories and flashbacks.

Life is a big thing with sex being one very important part of the whole. If sex goes wrong, it can spoil all of life for years to come.

Marriage is worth saving yourself for.

It really is worth the wait.

Joe S. McIlhaney Jr., an eminent gynecologist and popular speaker, is the author of *1,250 Health-Care Questions Women Ask* and co-author of *PMS: What It Is and What You Can Do about It*. He is currently president of the Medical Institute for Sexual Health (MISH) and devotes his time to promoting abstinence in public schools around the country.

Marion McIlhaney, Joe's wife, who taught high school English and worked as patient relations director at her husband's office, frequently speaks at women's retreats.